D e d i c a t i o n :

To my beloved children: Jean-Yves, Colette, Melanie, David-Benoît, Yahmeah, and Ezechiel, and stepchildren: Samuel and Adam.

Acknowledgements

Most scientists develop methods that improve over time through trial and error. The methods used in this book were conceived when I was a fellow in Allergy and Clinical Immunology at the Johns Hopkins Asthma and Allergy Center in Baltimore, Maryland. Over the years, through practice, my methods have much improved and many patients who have used them have enjoyed good health outcomes. I would therefore like to thank my patients from the University of Texas Health Sciences Center at Tyler (UTHSCT); those at the Center for Asthma, Allergy, Immunology & Hormone Health in Tyler, TX, and Woodbridge, VA; those at Fort Belvoir, VA; and finally, my current patients at Altru Health System, who have taught me so much and continue to reveal to me the etiology of allergic diseases and how to treat them. Those of you who have gone through my clinics and have seen the impact on your lives and have written to me about your satisfaction, I thank you for your useful comments, belief, and trust in me. I would like to thank my colleagues and the staff at Altru Health System, Fort Belvoir, and UTHSCT, who support my ideas and who are too many to list here, for their encouragements.

I would like to also thank the scientists at AhrQ for the HCUP data that provided solid evidence about allergic rhinitis, sinusitis, and conjunctivitis, and Bienvenue Tien, my nephew, who greatly helped in the making of the diagrams in this book.

I would like to thank my copy editor and proofreader Amberly Finarelli for her systematic line-by-line editing and her suggestions that have made this book a better finished product, and Stephanie Chandler and her team at Authority Publishing for their advice, encouragements, and efficient, timely production of this book.

Finally, I would like to thank Fatima, my wife and companion, who has continued to be my captive audience, for her patience, support, and love.

In the end, I must, as always, agree with Descartes that knowing that we know nothing is the beginning of real knowledge, and if knowledge comes from a higher power, then all thanks and praise should go to that higher power.

Benoît Tano, M.D., Ph.D.
Grand Forks, 2011

The
Allergy
Detective

Allergic Rhinitis Treatment Secrets
Your Doctor May Not Tell You

Benoît Tano, M.D., Ph.D.

The Allergy Detective: Allergic Rhinitis Treatment Secrets Your Doctor May Not Tell You

By Benoît Tano, M.D., Ph.D.

1. Health & Fitness : Diseases - Immune System 2. Health & Fitness : Alternative Therapies 3. Health & Fitness : Allergies

ISBN: 978-0-9834192-2-8

Library of Congress Control Number: 2011919777

Cover design by Lewis Agrell

Printed in the United States of America
Integrative Medical Press

Contents

INTRODUCTION 1

ALLERGIC RHINITIS, SINUSITIS,
AND CONJUNCTIVITIS ED DISCHARGES 5

ALLERGY IN CHILDHOOD 31

ESTROGEN EPIDEMIC AND ADULT-ONSET RHINITIS 39

SKIN TESTING AND ALLERGY VACCINE 49

MEDICATION THERAPY AND TREATMENT TECHNIQUES 63

OVERALL SUMMARY 73

APPENDIX A 77

BIBLIOGRAPHICAL NOTES..97

INDEX 139

ABOUT THE AUTHOR 145

Warning and disclaimer

Integrative Medical Press has designed this book to provide information about allergic rhinitis, perennial non-allergic rhinitis, sinusitis, and conjunctivitis. This information is derived from the author's practice of allergy and is not intended to replace your primary care physician or allergist. The publisher and the author are not liable for the misconception or misuse of the information provided in this book.

Every effort has been made to ensure that the information contained in this book is complete and accurate. The author and publisher assume neither liability nor responsibility to any person or entity with respect to any direct or indirect loss or damage caused, or alleged to be caused by the information contained herein, or for errors, omissions, inaccuracies, or any other inconsistency within these pages. The author has no conflict of interest to declare and does not have any financial interests and does not do any consulting or other business with the companies whose products are included in this book. The author is not promoting any particular products mentioned in this book.

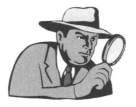 **INTRODUCTION**

Nose, eye, and sinus symptoms, commonly called allergies, fall under four major categories: allergic rhinitis (inflammation of the nasal membranes due to pollens, dust, dust mites, molds, pet dander, etc.), non-allergic rhinitis (inflammation of the nasal membranes due to chemicals — household cleaning agents, cigarette smoke, perfumes, flower scents, scented candles, air fresheners, petrochemicals, fumes, etc.), allergic conjunctivitis (inflammation of the eyes causing itchy, watery, puffy, swollen, red eyes), and sinusitis (acute and chronic sinus infections).

The bulk of allergy cases are treated by primary care health care providers. Many patients also self-treat, and the multiple over-the-counter (OTC) antihistamines available to the public attest to that. However, many health care providers do not have a deep understanding of the pathophysiology of rhinitis symptoms. Also, many patients who self-medicate use the weakest antihistamines, and often the more dangerous medications that lead to rhinitis medicamentosa (rebound nasal congestion), such as oxymetazoline (Afrin®). Others use nasal decongestants such as phenylephrine (Neo-Synephrine®) compounds and a combination of antihistamines and decongestants that can lead to high blood pressure. Understanding the mechanisms behind nasal symptoms and using an optimal combination of medications is necessary for effective treatment of nasal symptoms that are not benign. Untreated or poorly treated allergic and non-allergic rhinitis can lead to chronic and recurrent sinus infections, sinus pressure, headaches, and even asthma symptoms of chest tightness, shortness of breath, coughing, and wheezing. Postnasal drip, which is present in most allergy patients, is one of the most annoying, difficult-to-treat, and lingering rhinitis symptoms.

This guide, drawn from my own practice experience as an allergist, is intended to help all allergy sufferers take better control of their allergies. Health care professionals may also learn a brief pathophysiology of allergic and non-allergic rhinitis, as well as treatment protocols and techniques that will help their patients. In most cases of rhinitis, finding out the allergens by skin testing and desensitization by allergy vaccine leads to long-term relief, and qualified allergists (fellowship-trained allergists) will offer this service. If allergy sufferers are only interested in palliation (lessening) of their symptoms, they can often get good results by knowing what OTC medications work best and which ones to avoid. In this guide, you will learn about the medications that can give you relief, and how to save yourself money and grief.

Adult-onset nasal symptoms are on the rise, and are often frustrating for lack of understanding how to properly treat them. This guide explores the origins of this adult-onset allergy epidemic and the most effective ways to correct these symptoms. I will focus on both allergic and non-allergic rhinitis and their attendant derivatives of acute and chronic sinusitis, as well as allergic conjunctivitis. Chapter 1 presents rhinitis, sinusitis, and conjunctivitis statistics. In this chapter, the evidence of increasing allergic conditions is demonstrated by the emergency department (ED) discharges of these conditions for the year 2008, reported by the Healthcare Cost and Utilization Project (HCUP) data. This chapter opens a window to hormone imbalance that contributes to multiple pathological conditions prevalent in women, including rhinitis symptoms. Once the evidence is understood, the why, what, and how will be covered by understanding the pathophysiology of atopic diseases. The pathophysiology discussion is divided into two chapters: Chapter 2 presents allergy in childhood, and Chapter 3 presents the case of the estrogen epidemic and adult-onset rhinitis symptoms. The treatment of rhinitis begins with skin testing and an allergy vaccine, as discussed in Chapter 4, followed by medication therapy and treatment techniques, covered in Chapter 5. Finally, Chapter 6 offers some concluding remarks in an overall summary.

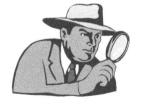

ALLERGIC RHINITIS, SINUSITIS, AND CONJUNCTIVITIS ED DISCHARGES

Allergic diseases are multiple and include:

- Allergic rhinitis
- Asthma
- Atopic dermatitis (eczema)
- Food allergy and anaphylaxis
- Drug allergy and anaphylaxis
- Urticaria and angioedema
- Sinusitis (which is a consequence of allergic and non-allergic rhinitis)
- Allergic conjunctivitis

This chapter covers rhinitis, sinusitis, and conjunctivitis from HCUP ED discharges data.

Tables 1-19, in Appendix A, present ED discharges for these allergic conditions for the year 2008 (U.S. only). The reported statistics seek to tease out the prevalence of allergic rhinitis, sinusitis, and conjunctivitis in women compared to men, and adults compared to children.

Summary

Tables 1-19 in Appendix A show that all cases of rhinitis, sinusitis, and conjunctivitis are more prevalent in women than in men. These allergic conditions are more prevalent in the 18-44 age groups. The South has the highest disease burden, followed by the Midwest, the Northeast, and the West. The increased disease burden in prime-age women may be due to hormone imbalance, until proven otherwise, and estrogen may be the culprit. The South and Midwest have the highest rates, possibly due to the high propensity of pesticides/herbicides used in farmlands in these two regions that lead to increased environmental estrogens.

Many of these conditions have high prevalence in women due to the increased endogenous estrogen production that couples with xenoestrogens (pesticides and herbicides, and the myriad of estrogenic products in cosmetics) and phytoestrogens (plant-based estrogens) to wreak havoc in women. This super-estrogen dominance in women manifests as the "multiple allergy" and other disease symptoms reported later on in this chapter. The next section will shed some light on the endogenous estrogen production process in men and women.

Sources of Endogenous Estrogens

Most endogenous estrogens in women are produced during the menstrual cycle but can also be produced by the adrenal glands and by conversion of testosterone to estrogen. Aromatase is the enzyme that facilitates the conversion of testosterone to estrogen. Obesity increases the activity of aromatase and hence, obese men and women tend to have more estrogens than lean individuals. Men produce estrogen by their bodies converting testosterone to estrogens via aromatase. Estrogen is responsible for the gynecomastia (man boobs) that men develop with increasing age, obesity, and alcohol abuse.

Estrogens in women and men are not benign, and the consequences will be covered in the following sections. The next section will cover the production of endogenous hormones.

Progesterone Deficiency, Estrogen Dominance, Leptin Resistance, Insulin Resistance, and Obesity

Our good hormones come from what is known as "bad" LDL cholesterol, which generates pregnenolone. Pregnenolone divides into two other hormones, progesterone and DHEA (DeHydroEpiAndrosterone); these two in turn produce estradiol, estrone, and testosterone. When we get older, we lose some of these hormones and others increase. The changes in hormones cause a hormonal disequilibrium, which is the source of many diseases and symptoms treated by health care providers. The diagram below is a rough illustration of endogenous hormone production cascade and consequences.

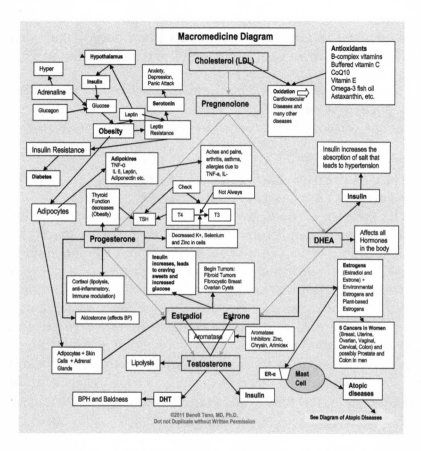

In this diagram, start with progesterone on the left: progesterone deficiency leads to increased estradiol and estrone, which lead to increased insulin. When insulin increases, initially glucose decreases, causing hypoglycemic episodes, and the individual often feels shaky and lightheaded. Adrenalin and glucagon therefore increase to augment the glucose level in the blood; insulin increase causes craving for sweets that also increase the glucose level.

Insulin then puts the excess glucose into adipocytes (fat cells) that cause obesity; filled adipocytes produce leptin to signal to the hypothalamus (center for satiety and craving) for decompression. The hypothalamus sends a message down to the insulin to stop the craving and reduce the appetite for weight loss; however, weight loss does not occur overnight — the adipocytes, not seeing the effect of their message to the hypothalamus, therefore continue to "complain" by producing more leptin. When the leptin message is too high, the hypothalamus ignores it and leptin resistance is created.

Leptin resistance causes a decrease in serotonin that leads to depression, anxiety, and panic attacks. Leptin resistance also leads to insulin resistance. Insulin resistance means that adipocytes shield themselves and do not want to absorb any more glucose. The glucose therefore remains in the blood and a high level creates what is called diabetes. The adipocytes also produce inflammatory cytokines such as TNF-α and IL-6 that cause aches and pains, arthritis, and allergic diseases such as asthma and rhinitis symptoms. The adipocytes also help the skin cells and adrenal glands to produce more estrogens (estradiol and estrone).

This endogenous increase in estrogens, coupled with environmental estrogens and plant-based estrogens, lead to benign tumors such as fibroid tumors, ovarian cysts, cervical dysplasia, fibrocystic breast disease in women, and benign prostatic hypertrophy (BPH) in men, and many other conditions. If you are not lucky and do not get a benign tumor, you may get a malignant tumor such as breast, uterine, ovarian, vaginal, cervical, or colon cancers in women and prostate or colon cancers in men. Estrogens have a receptor (binding site) on mast cells and basophils and when the estrogens attach to their receptor-alpha on these cells, the cells pour out histamine and leukotrienes just like pollens do.

Hence, increased estrogens not only directly increase allergies but also increase allergies through obesity. When progesterone decreases, thyroid function decreases, which leads to obesity. DHEA is the mother of all hormones. DHEA decreases with age and stress, which leads to insulin increase. Increase in insulin causes salt retention in kidney tubules that leads to hypertension. The decrease in DHEA therefore leads to obesity that eventually leads to allergic diseases, via increase in TNF-α and IL-6. The following will summarize the consequences of progesterone deficiency/estrogen dominance.

Progesterone Deficiency/Estrogen Dominance Creates a Chain Reaction

- Cortisol decrease (initially)
- Thyroid function decreases
- T4 does not always convert to T3
- TSH and free T4 may be in the "normal range" and free T3 may be low
- Measuring of TSH, free T4, and free T3 in a thyroid function test is therefore necessary
- Insulin increases
- Initially, hypoglycemia occurs
- Adrenaline is produced to increase glucose
- Glucagon is also produced to increase glucose
- Insulin causes an increase in carbohydrate consumption that leads to an increase in glucose
- Excess glucose is pushed into adipocytes by insulin

- Filled adipocytes produce leptin, adiponectin, visfatin, apelin
- Leptin signals to the hypothalamus that adipocytes are filled up
- The hypothalamus responds briefly, then stops when the demand is excessive
- Lack of response from the hypothalamus leads to leptin resistance
- Leptin resistance leads to a decrease in serotonin
- Decrease in serotonin leads to depression, anxiety, and panic attacks
- Leptin resistance also leads to insulin resistance
- Leptin and insulin resistance lead to type 2 diabetes
- Leptin resistance leads to increased ghrelin/NPY activities that lead to hunger and obesity
- Besides leptin and many other adipokines (chemicals used for communication by fat cells), adipocytes also make inflammatory cytokines such TNF-α and IL-6 that cause inflammation in the body such as arthritis, asthma, and allergic rhinitis
- Adipocytes help skin cells and adrenal glands to produce estradiol and estrone
- Estrogens increase both insulin and thyroid-binding globulin
- Increased thyroid-binding globulin further decreases thyroid function, which leads to more obesity
- Endogenous estrogens, environmental estrogens, and plant-based estrogens cause mast cells and basophils to release allergy-causing mediators that lead to allergy symptoms
- DHEA decreases with age and stress
- Decrease in DHEA causes insulin to increase

- Insulin increase causes salt retention that leads to hypertension
- Decrease in DHEA and progesterone lead to decreased testosterone
- Testosterone also converts to estrogens that lead to benign tumors, cancer, and allergic reactions
- When there is a hormone imbalance, the body tries to replenish the hormone by increasing the ingredient used to make the hormone
- Cholesterol — especially LDL cholesterol — increases so as to increase the production of the hormones
- Cholesterol is made in the liver and mixes with bile for better digestion of fat
- Sometimes bile salts are missing when the cholesterol gets to the gallbladder
- When bile salts are missing, the cholesterol precipitates and forms gallstones
- Gallstones block the common bile duct and therefore lead to inflammation of the gallbladder, called cholecystitis
- Cholecystitis leads to surgical removal of the gallbladder, called cholecystectomy
- In medical training, cholecystitis is known to be the disease of females, fat, fertile, and forty (the four F's)
- This condition is clearly related to hormone imbalance that occurs in women when they are in their 40s
- Decrease in progesterone and DHEA and increase in estradiol and estrone tend to increase insulin
- Progesterone modulates thyroid hormone activity by keeping potassium, zinc, and selenium in the cells. Potassium, zinc, and selenium are known to help convert T4 into T3 for increased metabolism

- Decrease in progesterone leads to estrogen dominance, and estrogen dominance leads to an increase in insulin and a further decrease in thyroid hormone activity. (Never rely on TSH alone as a thyroid function test. It is not uncommon to find elevated or decreased TSH level in the face of normal T4 and T3, and it is also common to find low free T3 in the face of normal free T4 and TSH.) It is also possible to see women on Synthroid with more weight problems, which suggests a suboptimal treatment of hypothyroidism.

Effects of Progesterone/Estrogen Imbalance on Women

This hormone imbalance creates:

- Premenstrual asthma (PMA)
- Premenstrual migraines
- Premenstrual dermatitis
- Non-allergic rhinitis and enhanced seasonal/perennial allergic rhinitis
- Fibromyalgia
- Menstrual disturbances
- Interstitial cystitis (IC), also known as overactive bladder. (IC is a mast-cell disease and is more prevalent in women than men; I suspect that estrogen dominance in women causes IC. When estrogen binds to its receptor-α on the mast cell, it causes mast cell degranulation in the detrusor muscle of the bladder that leads to the IC symptoms. Hence, balancing estrogen by giving adequate amounts of progesterone and DIM or I-3-C may help IC patients.)
- Arthritis

- Non-allergic rhinitis and seasonal/perennial allergic rhinitis
- Obesity and asthma

What do obesity and asthma have in common? They are both influenced by estrogen.

Progesterone Deficiency and Consequences

Both men and women produce progesterone. While progesterone is produced by the adrenal glands and testes in men, progesterone in women is produced during the menstrual cycle by the ovaries and adrenal glands. The low progesterone gene can be inherited from the mother, and low progesterone in the mother can lead to low progesterone in the daughter or son.

When girls inherit the low progesterone gene, they developed progesterone deficiency symptoms early in life. Right after menarche (onset of menstrual periods), the young girl starts experiencing menorrhagia (heavy menstrual periods) and/or dysmenorrhea (painful menstrual cramps), often accompanied by nausea, vomiting, and diarrhea. This is quite debilitating for many young girls. These women also often have difficulty conceiving and if they conceive, they have difficulty carrying the pregnancy to term. They tend to have multiple miscarriages, and if an astute OB/GYN physician realizes the low progesterone problem and injects even synthetic progesterone, the pregnancy can go to term.

If the low-progesterone woman becomes pregnant, the first trimester could represent a real challenge. She will have nausea and vomiting throughout the pregnancy, but these symptoms are worse in the first trimester when the progesterone production is still average. During the second trimester, the placenta produces about 400 mg of progesterone a day, and that helps resolve the nausea and vomiting problem. After delivery, when the placenta is gone, the progesterone production decreases to average and the woman becomes depressed. This may explain much of the postpartum depression experienced by many women. The low progesterone also causes many symptoms, and many of these symptoms are the same as estrogen dominance because estrogen dominance is simply normal or high estrogen in the face of low progesterone.

Adult-Onset Progesterone Deficiency

If a woman does not have low progesterone to begin with, as she gets older she tends to lose her progesterone because of anovulatory menstrual cycles (menstrual cycles without ovulation). Women also lose their progesterone because of progesterone-containing birth control pills (progestins) that suppress the natural production of progesterone. Women produce progesterone during their menstrual cycle as follows:

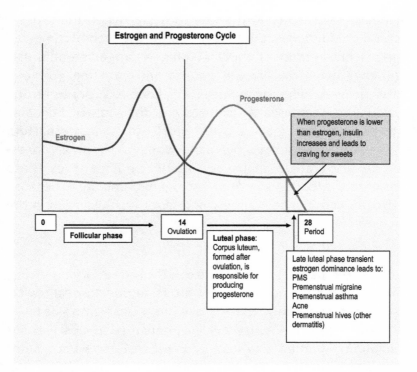

Progesterone is produced after ovulation. In women who have a normal cycle of 28 days, the 14th day is known as ovulation or when the egg (ovum) is released from the ovary. When the egg is released, the pocket where the egg came from does not disappear. It becomes yellow and is known as the "yellow body," or corpus luteum in Latin. The female menstrual cycle is therefore divided into three phases: pre-ovulatory phase or follicular phase, ovulatory phase, and post-ovulatory phase, also known as the luteal phase because of the activity of the corpus luteum. Before ovulation, the estrogens estradiol and estrone increase, reach their peak around ovulation time, and decline thereafter. Progesterone is flat prior to ovulation, but right after ovulation it starts to increase and peaks about seven days before a woman's period. Three to five days (but sometimes a week) before the period, many women develop premenstrual syndrome (PMS) or premenstrual dysphoric disorder (PMDD).

PMS and PMDD can consist of an uneasy feeling, emotional lability, bloating, acne, premenstrual asthma exacerbations for post-pubertal women with asthma, premenstrual migraines, premenstrual dermatitis (hives), and most women around the world crave sweets — chocolate is only one of them. The sugar craving is due to the activity of insulin, which is the sugar-craving hormone. Insulin increases when progesterone decreases below estrogen in the last week of the menstrual cycle. This transient insulin increase is responsible for the sugar craving.

Women tend to have anovulatory menstrual cycles in their late 20s, early 30s, mid-30s, and beyond. This leads to progressive dwindling of the protective hormone progesterone, and the ensuing unopposed estrogen leads to a persistent, instead of transient, insulin increase. This permanent insulin increase in turn leads to constant craving for sweets. Eating sweets or high-sugar-content foods leads to increase in blood glucose. The insulin has to quickly dispose of the glucose so as to prevent it from spilling in the blood. The quickest way of getting rid of the glucose in the blood is to put it into the fat cells. Fat cells convert the glucose into fatty acids for storage and the end result is obesity. Hence, it is not surprising to see women gain weight after age 35, or even sooner if their progesterone deficiency starts earlier.

When progesterone decreases, thyroid function also decreases, which compounds the weight gain problem.

How does thyroid function connect to progesterone? Progesterone aids in the retention of zinc, potassium, and selenium in our cells. Zinc, potassium, and selenium allow the thyroid hormone T4 to enter the cell and then to be converted to the active form T3 that is used for metabolism. Low progesterone decreases this mineral retention in cells. As a result, T4 does not convert to T3. Patients with hypothyroidism are given a T4 equivalent: levothyroxine (Synthroid). If the patient has low progesterone, as occurs in menopausal women, then this treatment remains ineffective. These patients do not readily lose the weight and if T3 is measured, it is found to be low. T3 may be within the standardized specified range that no one should deviate from, but on the low end of the range. The TSH in this case is often greater than 2. If 0.49-4.47 is the normal range, and 0.49 is considered perfectly optimal thyroid function, then anything above 0.49 is not perfect. Anything above this perfect number is signaling that the body needs a little more thyroid to optimally achieve metabolism. Unfortunately, the rigid standard of care does not even consider a patient's possible symptoms of continued fatigue and difficulty in losing weight despite the thyroid supplementation. Patients continue to be treated with the same medications, even though the results are not there. This leads to frustration, and patients seek alternative therapies on their own.

Increased estrogen leads to increased thyroid binding globulin that binds both T4 and T3 tightly and does not relinquish them for metabolism. Some scientists have therefore suggested that women be supplemented with thyroid medication when they are on birth control pills. Birth control pills prevent ovulation and therefore decrease the progesterone level in the users. Hence, many women on these pills tend to gain weight.

Estrogen is also associated with copper. Copper is required for the synthesis and release of estrogen and also forms enzymes in the liver, which help to break down leftover estrogen into harmless substances. Estrogen can cause copper retention if zinc or progesterone levels are too low or calcium level is high. Since copper contributes to the increase in estrogen, an increase in copper level in the body may therefore decrease thyroid function.

If calcium and copper increase together, they can have a detrimental effect on thyroid function. By antagonizing estrogen and allowing potassium, selenium, and zinc to remain in cells, progesterone reverses all these negative mineral effects on thyroid function. Unfortunately, TSH, measured by most physicians to test for thyroid function, often does not capture this imbalance.

Estrogens also cause benign tumors in women as mentioned above. In men, prostate enlargement, called benign prostatic hypertrophy, may be due to too much estrogen. This condition is usually linked to dihydrotestosterone, a more potent form of testosterone, blamed for causing male pattern baldness and prostate enlargement.

Estrogens, Benign Tumors, and Many Other Conditions in Women

- Fibroid tumors
- Fibrocystic breast disease

- Ovarian cysts
- Cervical dysplasia (non-HPV related)
- Endometriosis

Estrogens and Cancer

- Studies of estrogen metabolism have led to the hypothesis that reaction of certain estrogen metabolites, predominantly catechol estrogen-3,4-quinones with DNA, can generate the critical mutations initiating breast, prostate, and other cancers.
- The endogenous estrogens estrone (E1) and estradiol (E2) are oxidized to catechol estrogens (CE), 2- and 4-hydroxylated estrogens, which can be further oxidized to CE quinones that are involved in breast and prostate cancers.

Estrogen is associated with the following cancers and perhaps many more:

- Breast cancer
- Uterine cancer
- Ovarian cancer
- Cervical cancer
- Vaginal cancer
- Colon cancer
- Prostate cancer

Estrogen and Progesterone Receptors in Breast Cancer

- ER (estrogen-receptor) positive/PR (progesterone-receptor) positive (this type of breast cancer is more prevalent than other types of breast cancer)

- ER positive/PR negative
- ER negative/PR positive
- ER negative/PR negative

Estrogenic Chemicals and Allergic Diseases: The Case of BPA

A 2010 study on mice has concluded that perinatal exposure to 10 micrograms/mL of BPA in drinking water enhances allergic sensitization and bronchial inflammation and responsiveness in an animal model of asthma (adult-onset allergies due to estrogen dominance will be covered in Chapter 3).

Endocrine Disrupting Chemicals, Hormone Imbalance, and Diseases in Humans

Women tend to produce more estrogens from their late 20s on. Most women become estrogen dominant because their endogenous production of estrogens increases when they lose their progesterone due to anovulatory menstrual cycles. Women who go on birth control pills tend to develop hormone disruption sooner. Increased endogenous estrogens, coupled with environmental estrogens (xenoestrogens and phytoestrogens), lead to multiple symptoms that women present with to their doctors. Unfortunately, since there is no true training in hormone disruption and correction of its ill effects in medical schools or residency programs, and since most endocrinologists are busy dealing with diabetes, thyroid diseases, and more familiar endocrine conditions, there are few physicians who will touch these symptoms. The few physicians who try to investigate these conditions do well by helping these patients. However, since most medical professionals are not well versed in the literature regarding the effects of endocrine disruptors, they pose as judges of the few who try to find solutions.

What Causes Estrogen Dominance?

- Endogenous estrogens
- Exogenous estrogens

Xenoestrogens: herbicides, pesticides, and other household chemicals, including cosmetics and cosmeceuticals.

Phytoestrogens: Plant estrogens such as found in bay leaf, celery, nutmeg, cloves, cinnamon, alfalfa sprouts, cottonseed oil, cumin, tea, tea tree oil, oregano, Melaleuca products, dates, thyme, peppermint, turmeric, fenugreek, feverfew, pomegranate, flax oil, wheat (weak phytoestrogen), garlic, hemp oil, red clover, hops (beer), rosemary, caffeine, coffee (including decaffeinated coffee), safflower, safflower oil, canola oil, chamomile, chamomile tea, licorice, soy, chocolate and its main product cocoa, clover, mint, sunflower oil, sunflower seeds, only to name a few. (See additional xenoestrogens and phytoestrogens listed by Peter Eckhart, M.D., at www.woomhoo.com.)

Progesterone deficiency and estrogen dominance therefore lead to multiple pathological conditions treated by health care professionals.

Some of these progesterone/estrogen imbalance symptoms are:

- Abdominal bloating
- Absence of maternal instinct and behavior
- Acne
- Agitation
- Agoraphobia
- Alcohol abuse
- Allergies or sensitivities to foods or chemicals
- Allergy shiners in adults (dark circles under the eyes)
- Anovulatory menstrual cycles
- Anxiety
- Asthma
- Binges
- Blood clots
- Breast and/or ovarian cysts
- Breast tenderness
- Brown patches on cheeks
- Brown spots on backs of hands
- Bruising and capillary breakage
- Burning eyes
- Carbohydrate cravings
- Chronic fatigue
- Claustrophobia
- Clumsiness
- Cold hands and feet
- Constipation
- Cracked heels
- Cravings for sweets
- Depression
- Depression after childbirth
- Depression during peri-menopause/menopause

- Difficulty in getting up after enough sleep
- Dizziness
- Dry skin
- Dysmenorrhea (painful menstrual cramps)
- Early aging of skin
- Early miscarriages
- Emotionally labile (easy crying, quick to anger)
- Endometriosis
- Excessive facial and body hair on women
- Exhaustion
- Fainting spells
- Feelings of aggression
- Feelings of guilt
- Feelings of insecurity
- Feelings of loneliness
- Feelings of resentment
- Feelings of tension
- Feelings of unreality
- Feelings of uselessness, worthlessness
- Fibroid tumors
- Flaking, brittle, and weak nails
- Follicular keratoses ("goose bumps") on backs of arms and legs
- Forgetting what you're about to say — mental block
- Frequent complaining
- Frequent or regular headaches
- Frequent or regular migraines
- Foggy thinking
- Hallucinations
- Histrionic behavior
- Hot flashes/flushes
- Hypoglycemia

- Inability to concentrate
- Incontinence
- Infanticide fears
- Infertility
- Infertility/difficulty in becoming pregnant
- Insomnia
- Internally upset by criticism
- Irrational fears
- Irregular menstrual flow
- Irregular periods
- Irritability
- Itching skin
- Lack of menstrual periods
- Lack of self-confidence and self-esteem
- Lethargy
- Loss of libido
- Low blood pressure
- Low libido
- Lower body temperature
- Maltreatment of newborn baby; harmful, violent thoughts
- Manic behavior
- Manic/depressive (bipolar disorder)
- Menorrhagia
- Miscarriages
- Misty vision
- Mood swings
- Nausea during pregnancy
- Nervousness
- Night sweats
- Obsessions without compulsions
- Osteoporosis

- Ovarian cysts
- Painful eyes
- Palpitations
- Panic attacks or panicky feelings
- Paranoia
- PCOS (polycystic ovarian syndrome)
- Period pains and/or ovulation cramps
- Personality changes
- Pre-eclampsia
- Premenstrual backache
- Premenstrual breast tenderness
- Procrastination
- Prostate problems
- Puffiness/bloating
- Quick reaction or overreaction to alcohol
- Quick-tempered
- Rage
- Regular epileptic fits not due to brain injury
- Rejection of baby
- SAD (seasonal affective disorder)
- Self-mutilation
- Sense of confusion
- Shaking or trembling
- Short-term memory loss
- Sleep disturbances
- Spaced out
- Suicidal thoughts or attempts
- Temporary psychosis
- Thinning of hair/hair loss (women)
- Tired all the time
- Tricotilomania (hair pulling)
- Vaginal thinning, dryness, and itching

- Varicose veins
- Verbal and physical violence
- Water retention
- Weight gain at puberty/childbirth/menopause

Laboratory Workup

When you suspect hormone imbalance, you should order tests for progesterone, DHEA, DHEA-S, androstenedione, estradiol, estrone, cortisol, aldosterone (if patient has hypertension or hypotension), fasting insulin, leptin level (if patient is obese), lipid panel, comprehensive metabolic panel, total and free testosterone, dihydrotestosterone (DHT), sex hormone binding globulin (SHBG), FSH and LH, homocysteine, high sensitivity CRP, TSH, free T4 and free T3, Somatomedin-C (IGF-1), and IGFBP3. These tests should be ordered for both men and women, adding PSA for men.

The laboratory test that will accurately measure the part of LDL (oxidized LDL) that causes plaque formation in the arteries is currently available in some laboratories. It is important to look at the proportion of LDL that is oxidized because that portion is what is dangerous, and LDL does not have to be elevated to oxidize. Remember that LDL is needed for production of steroid hormones. Hence, lowering total LDL may be detrimental to the body. Preventing oxidation of LDL using antioxidants makes more sense.

Hormone Imbalance Types

Based on my clinical evaluation of patients who present with hormone imbalance, the laboratory results show 12 different hormonal patterns. The first group has no deficiency and there are very few of these individuals. The second group only lacks progesterone; the third group lacks both progesterone and estradiol; the fourth group lacks progesterone, estradiol, and DHEA. The fifth group lacks progesterone, estradiol, DHEA, and testosterone. Those individuals also often lack pregnenolone. You can follow through the table and see all the possible hormone deficiency combinations.

Progesterone	Estradiol	DHEA	Testosterone
+	+	+	+
-	+	+	+
-	-	+	+
-	-	-	+
-	-	-	-
+	+	+	-
+	-	-	-
+	-	-	-
+	+	+	-
+	-	-	+
-	-	-	+
-	+	+	-

This chapter has demonstrated that the endogenous production of hormones leads to estrogen dominance that couples with environmental estrogens and plant-based estrogens to cause multiple pathological conditions. Women with increased endogenous estrogens therefore will experience the bulk of estrogen-related conditions, including allergic reactions. The growing incidence of adult-onset allergic reactions and the evidence obtained by the HCUP database on allergic rhinitis, sinusitis, and conjunctivitis attest to that.

The next two chapters will present the pathophysiology (mechanisms) behind the observed allergic diseases.

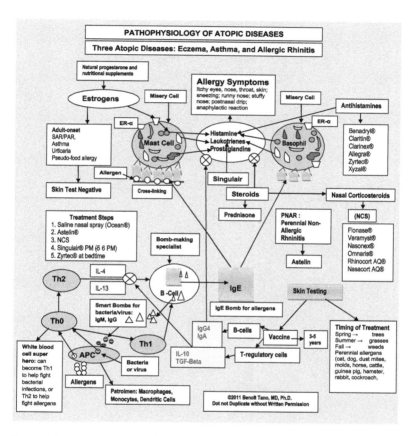

The pathophysiology of atopic diseases is different in children than in many adults. Chapter 2 presents allergy in childhood, and Chapter 3 presents adult-onset allergy.

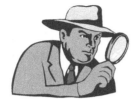

ALLERGY IN CHILDHOOD

For some individuals, allergies start in childhood. These individuals tend to inherit the genes from one or both of their parents. If one parent has allergies, the child has about a 40% chance of developing allergies; if both parents have allergies, the child has about a 70% to 90% chance of developing allergies. The allergy gene alone does not cause allergic reactions. To react, the individual has to have the gene and be in the right environment. Gene-environmental interactions lead to allergic reactions. The prevalence of allergic diseases in the developed world is partially explained by the hygiene hypothesis, which holds that allergies are due to too much cleanliness. In developing countries, people's immune systems are busy fighting widespread bacteria and have no time to concentrate on innocuous substances such as pollens and other allergens. However, in the developed world where individuals are not much exposed to bacteria, the immune system, looking for work, turns to fighting these innocuous substances.

There are three diseases that go together and are known

collectively as atopic diseases: atopic dermatitis (eczema), asthma, and allergic rhinitis. There is something called the atopic march, which is a progression of atopic diseases in which children start with eczema around age 4 months to 5 months, when they are first exposed to solid foods. By age 3 months to 4 months, sometimes sooner and other times later, some of the children develop upper respiratory infections, such as respiratory syncytial virus (RSV) infection and other viral infections that lead to their first wheeze (asthma symptoms). These symptoms, often called reactive airway disease by many primary care physicians, may continue until adulthood, or may subside early in childhood. By age 2, most children with atopy have developed their allergic rhinitis symptoms. Sometimes, the sequence is eczema-allergic rhinitis-asthma, or asthma-eczema-allergic rhinitis. If the children develop allergic rhinitis that is untreated or poorly treated, they can develop asthma symptoms as a consequence; this is known as allergic rhinitis impact on asthma (ARIA).

Food allergy is a fourth condition that may go along with these three atopic diseases. It often contributes to the exacerbations of atopic dermatitis, and when that is discovered, elimination of the food from the child's diet helps alleviate the atopic dermatitis symptoms. The five most common foods that cause allergy in children are peanut, soy, milk, egg, and wheat.

Chronic sinusitis is a consequence of a poorly treated rhinitis. When the mucus does not drain from the sinuses, it becomes a breeding ground for bacteria that leads to a sinus infection called sinusitis. Acute sinusitis may be caused by a viral infection and therefore may not respond to antibiotics; it may simply have to run its course. It is therefore important to observe an acute sinusitis for about seven days prior to initiating an antibiotic therapy. I will show you how to prevent acute sinusitis in Chapter 5.

In order to react to allergens, the individual has to be sensitized. The process of sensitization starts with exposure of the allergens to an antigen-presenting cell (APC), such as macrophages, monocytes, dendritic cells, or B cells, that I call the "patrolmen." The APC then presents the allergens to Th0 cells that I call "white blood cell super heroes," because they can differentiate into Th2 cells or Th1 cells. Th1 cells are specialized in stimulating B cells (bomb-making specialists) to produce antibodies (smart bombs called IgM and IgG) for fighting bacteria, viruses, and other non-allergic infectious pathogens.

Upon exposure to allergens, the APC's signal to the Th0 cell, which transforms into a Th2 cell. Once the Th2 cells are formed, they produce IL-4 and IL-13 (interleukins 4 and 13, which are chemicals used by Th2 cells to communicate — view these chemicals as the Th2's cell phones) that stimulate the B cells to produce IgE (a smart bomb for fighting allergens). The B cell is so versatile that it can produce IgE against all allergens (tree, grass, and weed pollens, dust mites, molds, animal dander, cockroach, etc.). If you view the IgE as a bomb, this bomb does not explode until it attaches to its docking sites, known as IgE receptors.

Once the IgE is formed, it circulates in the blood and finds its receptors on two white blood cells: mast cells that live in the skin and tissues, and basophils that circulate in blood vessels with other blood cells. These two cells have the IgE receptor called FCεR1 (spelled "FC epsilon receptor 1" — you do not have to remember this receptor name and I promise, there will be no quiz on it). Once the IgE finds its receptors, it binds them. At that point, these "misery cells," as I call mast cells and basophils because they make millions of people miserable around the world, are armed, dangerous, and waiting for the next encounter to explode.

When an individual is exposed to the same allergen again, the allergen goes through the nose, eventually makes its way to the blood system, and finds the specific IgE's that are already on the surface of the misery cells and binds them. A cross-linking of the IgE-antigen molecules occurs, and that is a signal for these misery cells to pour out their preformed granules in a process called degranulation. The first chemical granule that is released is histamine. Histamine is a nerve-ending irritant and causes itching. The individual therefore experiences itchy eyes, itchy nose, itchy throat, sneezing, runny nose, and sometimes, itchy skin.

To treat these symptoms, antihistamines such as Benadryl®, Claritin®, Clarinex®, Allegra®, Zyrtec®, and Xyzal® are given. Zyrtec®, which became available over-the-counter in 2008, is one of the best antihistamines. Allegra®, also very good, is now over-the-counter. What I often see in my practice is that patients tend to go for the weakest antihistamines, such as Benadryl® and Claritin®, first and rarely try Zyrtec® or Allegra® first. However, though I generally prescribe Zyrtec® or Allegra®, this recommendation may not be optimal for everyone. I have seen a few patients who actually had better results with Claritin® or Benadryl®. These patients have tried either Zyrtec® or Allegra® and did not get any positive results. Other patients tried Zyrtec®, which led to drowsiness, and therefore they used Claritin®, which is milder, and it worked better for them. This means that in allergy treatment, one size does not fit all. If you try the more potent antihistamines and you are having problems or you are not getting any relief, try one of the other antihistamines listed above. Individuals who need to stay awake, such as pilots or air traffic controllers, should use Allegra® instead of Zyrtec®.

If histamine were the only chemical released by mast cells and basophils, the allergy solution would be simple: use antihistamines and there will be no more symptoms. However, there are many other chemicals produced by these misery cells. Two of these chemicals, leukotrienes C4 (LTC4) and prostaglandins, tend to cause late-phase allergic reactions: stuffy nose, postnasal drip, coughing, and for asthmatics, constriction of the airways and therefore, wheezing. One other cell, eosinophil, releases chemicals that are also involved in the late-phase reaction. The symptoms mentioned above tend to occur at night for most allergy and asthma sufferers because the leukotrienes are produced at night. To block the leukotrienes, montelukast (which is available as a medication known as Singulair®), the most popular leukotriene receptor antagonist (LTRA) was conceived, along with other leukotriene receptor antagonists.

Children and adults who have allergic rhinitis and asthma symptoms should therefore use a combination of a good antihistamine, such as Zyrtec® or Allegra®, and a good LTRA, such as Singulair®. This combination therapy will, in most cases, be optimal. The mistake made by most patients who self-treat and by primary care providers is trying these medications one at a time; many people first try antihistamines only, and if they do not get good relief, they switch to LTRA. This stepwise approach to allergy treatment is not effective. Advil® Cold and Sinus works to block the prostaglandins, hence ibuprofen in general can block prostaglandins.

The master blocker of all these chemicals released by the misery cells are steroids, which is why many health care providers inject steroids or give prednisone to their patients when they present with allergy symptoms. Systemic steroids, however, have multiple undesirable side effects in both adults and children and should be reserved only for short-term bursts for brittle asthma or other severe atopic inflammation. For the treatment of allergic rhinitis, nasal corticosteroids (NCS's) that act locally are desirable, and they include:

- Flonase® (fluticasone), which is now generic: approved for ages 4 and older.
- Veramyst® (fluticasone): also approved for ages 4 and older.
- Nasonex®: most desirable for children and is approved for ages 2 and older.
- Omnaris® (ceclosenide): approved for ages 6 and older.
- Rhinocort AQ® (budesonide): approved for ages 6 and older, and pregnant women with allergies.
- Nasacort AQ® (triamcinolone): approved for ages 6 and older.

Treatment for allergic diseases therefore requires a combination therapy: antihistamines to block the histamine released from mast cells and basophils, LTRA to block the leukotrienes, and NCS's to block all the chemicals that participate in allergic reactions. The effective use of these medications will be covered in Chapter 5.

The allergy theory stipulates that allergies start in childhood. However, more and more adults and especially women, as demonstrated by the HCUP data in Chapter 1, are presenting to my clinic and other medical offices with adult-onset nasal symptoms. Chapter 3 will shed some light on this phenomenon.

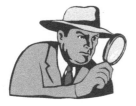

ESTROGEN
EPIDEMIC AND
ADULT-ONSET
RHINITIS

As mentioned in Chapter 2, allergies start in childhood. However, in my practice, I am seeing more and more patients who present in adulthood (ages 15 and older) with complaints of nasal symptoms, asthma symptoms, severe urticaria (hives)/angioedema (lips, tongue, facial or whole body swelling), and even newly acquired food allergies (that I call pseudo-food allergy), such as shellfish and nut allergies.

Recent CDC reports about atopic diseases seem to point to a growing allergy problem in women, and obesity and estrogens are hinted at as possible culprits. Several articles listed by the American Academy of Allergy, Asthma and Immunology (AAAAI) website have implicated obesity and even touched on hormone imbalance as culprits of the growing allergy epidemic. As an allergist who sees manifestation of allergic diseases in pediatric and adult patients, I have also come to conclude that the growing atopy in American adults is due to an estrogen epidemic, which is neither fully investigated nor understood. In the next ten years, the evidence supporting my conclusions may become clearer. The next section will look at atopic diseases as windows to the whole body, and will point out the estrogen connection to many of the atopic diseases treated by allergists.

Estrogens and Mast Cell Response

The HCUP data analysis reported in Chapter 1 points to higher levels of adult-onset allergic rhinitis in women than in men. Why are women so vulnerable to this allergy epidemic? The following analysis will attempt to provide some answers to this question.

Recently, research conducted by professor Midoro-Horiuti and colleagues at the University of Texas Medical Branch (UTMB) in Galveston, Texas, and appearing in *Environmental Health Perspectives* 115:48-52 (2007), demonstrated that estradiol activates mast cells (remember our misery cells?) via an estrogen receptor-alpha(ER-α) on these mast cells and calcium influx. The research demonstrated that estradiol alone induced partial release of the preformed granular protein β-hexosaminidase from RBL-2H3 (see definition in bibliographical notes), BMMC (bone marrow-derived mast cell), and HMC-1(human mast cell line), but not from BMMC derived from estrogen receptor-α knock-out mice (mice that lack the estrogen receptor-alpha). The newly synthesized leukotriene C4 (LTC4) was also released from RBL-2H3. Estradiol also enhanced IgE-induced degranulation and potentiated LTC4 production. Intracellular calcium concentration increased prior to and in parallel with mediator release. Estrogen receptor antagonists or calcium$^+$ chelation inhibited these estrogenic effects.

They concluded that binding of physiological concentrations of estradiol to a membrane estrogen receptor-α initiates a rapid onset and progressive influx of extracellular calcium, which supports the synthesis and release of allergic mediators. Estradiol also enhances IgE-dependent mast cell activation, resulting in a shift of the allergen dose response.

The same research group examined the effects of environmental pollutants that have estrogen-like activities and are termed environmental estrogens (for example, DDT, endosulfan, atrazine, and many thousands more used as pesticides and herbicides in agriculture) in allergic diseases. These pollutants tend to degrade slowly in the environment and to bioaccumulate and bioconcentrate in the food chain; they also have long biological half-lives.

The goal in this study was to identify possible pathogenic roles for environmental estrogens in the development of allergic diseases. They screened a number of environmental estrogens for their ability to modulate the release of allergic mediators from mast cells. They incubated a human mast cell line and primary mast cell cultures derived from bone marrow of wild type and estrogen receptor-α (ER-α)-deficient mice with environmental estrogens with and without estradiol or IgE and allergens. They then assessed degranulation of mast cells by quantifying the release of beta-hexosaminidase (a mast cell product).

The results showed that all the environmental estrogens tested caused rapid, dose-related release of beta-hexosaminidase from mast cells and enhanced IgE-mediated release. The combination of physiologic concentrations of 17-β-estradiol and several concentrations of environmental estrogens had additive effects on mast cell degranulation. Comparison of bone marrow mast cells from ER-α-sufficient and ER-α-deficient mice indicated that much of the effect of environmental estrogens was mediated by ER-α. They concluded that their findings suggest that estrogenic environmental pollutants might promote allergic diseases by inducing and enhancing mast cell degranulation by physiologic estrogens and exposure to allergens.

In reference to the UTMB studies reported above, it is now well-known that mast cells have a high-affinity ER-α. Binding of your own estrogens (estradiol and estrone) and estrogens produced by agrichemicals and household chemicals, including cosmetics and cosmeceuticals, to this receptor induce mast cell degranulation, with release of histamine and LTC4 that cause the allergy symptoms.

I generally inform adult-onset-allergy patients that their allergy symptoms may not be related to usual environmental allergens. Since these patients are convinced that they have seasonal/perennial allergic rhinitis, I always offer a skin testing, and patients are often surprised to see that their skin-testing results are negative. Others are in disbelief and even think that the skin test is faulty. I couple the test with a measure of the patient's endogenous hormones, and in most cases the estrogen is too high and the progesterone too low. I have been able to give bioidentical progesterone (progesterone identical to what the body makes) to these patients and their allergy symptoms often improve.

Since xenoestrogens and phytoestrogens play a major role

in adult-onset allergic processes, I give the patients a list of xenoestrogens and phytoestrogens to avoid. I also recommend nutritional supplements that help with their overall well-being. Many of these patients suffering from adult-onset asthma, steroid-dependent dermatitis (such as hives), or perennial non-allergic rhinitis (chemical sensitivity), also have important comorbidities, such as obesity, hypothyroidism, hyperlipidemia, hypertension, insulin resistance, and female menstrual disturbances such as menstrual irregularity, fibroid tumors with menorrhagia (heavy menstrual bleeding), metrorrhagia (uterine bleeding at irregular intervals, particularly between the expected menstrual periods), menometrorrhagia (excessive uterine bleeding, both at the usual time of menstrual periods and at other irregular intervals), fibrocystic breast disease, ovarian cysts, and endometriosis. Often, these patients have seen multiple physicians for these conditions. Some have had a hysterectomy, while others have had breast biopsies that have revealed fibrocystic breast disease. Many of these women are on birth control pills to control their menstrual problems; many others are on antidepressants for depression, panic attacks, nervousness, and anxiety. Chronic chest pain due to anxiety is often seen in patients who have been evaluated by cardiologists, and in some cases cardiac catheterization has been performed without any findings. Many of these patients have high cholesterol and high blood pressure and are therefore on cholesterol and blood-pressure-lowering medications.

These patients most often have estrogen dominance. Estrogen dominance, by definition, is normal or high estrogen in presence of deficient progesterone. The excess estrogens, coupled with environmental estrogens and plant-based estrogens (such

as soy, hops in beer, wheat), cause allergic disease by stimulating the estrogen receptors on the mast cells, and also by
potentiating the effect of IgE antibody (remember the effect
of the IgE bomb produced by the B cells?) on the mast cells,
and estrogen receptors on basophils, to release histamine
and LTC4. The degranulation of these mast cells and basophils
tend to release products that are responsible for many allergic
reactions — nasal symptoms being just part of the allergy
conundrum.

One situation that occurs often is the anaphylactic reaction to
allergen immunotherapy (AIT), which is also more common
in women than in men. I recently saw a woman who was on
AIT and could not reach maintenance because of anaphylactic
reactions. I reformulated her AIT extracts and started her
on a slower injection schedule. She was able to go through
the yellow vial, and on her second dose of the red vial (the
concentrate antigen) she had another anaphylactic reaction.
This time, instead of simply reformulating her AIT extracts or
changing her injection schedule, I measured her hormones
and, not surprisingly, her estrogen level was very high and
progesterone level very low. I started her on progesterone and
continued her on her AIT. She was also having unexplained
syncope episodes and these symptoms resolved when she
started on the progesterone therapy. In this case, the high
endogenous estrogen caused a synergistic effect with the
IgE on the mast cells that led to her recurrent anaphylactic
reactions. Since this case, I have seen three more young
women who had similar episodes. The most recent case of
anaphylaxis occurred in my clinic in October 2010. The young
woman was in day 12 or 13 of her pre-ovulation menstrual
phase, which is usually characterized by high estrogen level

(see estrogen and progesterone cycle diagram below).

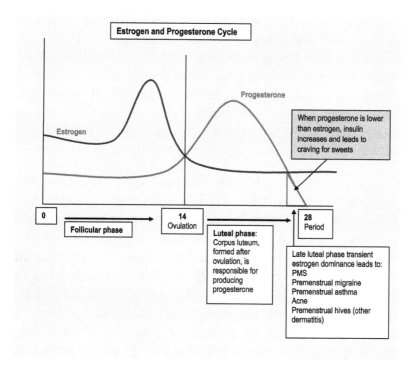

Estrogen and Progesterone Cycle

Estrogen

Progesterone

When progesterone is lower than estrogen, insulin increases and leads to craving for sweets

| 0 | 14 Ovulation | 28 Period |

Follicular phase

Luteal phase: Corpus luteum, formed after ovulation, is responsible for producing progesterone

Late luteal phase transient estrogen dominance leads to: PMS Premenstrual migraine Premenstrual asthma Acne Premenstrual hives (other dermatitis)

She had an anaphylactic reaction to her AIT injection. I have since recommended that she skip her AIT injections in her pre-ovulatory phase and three to five days before onset of her menstrual period, which also corresponds to a transient estrogen dominance state (estrogen greater than progesterone). I have also started her on low-dose progesterone because her measured estrogen was elevated and her progesterone was low (remember that high estrogen causes mast cells to pour out their chemical granules, such as histamines and leukotrienes, that cause allergic reactions). She has since not had any more episodes, and she has tolerated her AIT injections and reached maintenance.

In several cases if a patient reacts several times to the AIT injections, to avoid any potential liability the patient is told to stop the AIT. Allergists should therefore take into account estrogen dominance and phytoestrogens' and xenoestrogens' effects when evaluating patients suspected of adult-onset allergies and AIT-induced anaphylactic reactions. When the actual cause of the symptoms is discovered and treated, both the patient and the allergist are rewarded.

The cases of skin test reactivity variation with the phases of the menstrual cycle (see Nelson, *Immunology and Allergy Clinics of North America*, 2001 and Kalogeromitros, et al., *Clinical Experimental Allergy*, 1995) and premenstrual asthma (late luteal phase asthma exacerbations) in women (see Nakasato, et al., *Journal of Asthma*, 1999) are well-documented in the allergy literature. However, allergists do not routinely take this into account in their practices when doing skin testing and when women react to AIT. In the case of premenstrual asthma, Nakasato, et al., recommended Singulair® as a good treatment. It is clear that in the late luteal phase, progesterone falls below estrogen (see diagram above), and that transient estrogen dominance is responsible for making the mast cells highly responsive (twicky) and for causing premenstrual asthma or premenstrual exacerbations of allergy symptoms in premenopausal women. In these cases, LTC4 is released in addition to histamine, and therefore a combination of antihistamines and Singulair® (LTRA) is optimal.

Since learning about hormones and their relationship to allergic reaction, I have been able to pinpoint the actual culprits in these so-called adult-onset allergies.

Another cause of adult-onset rhinitis independent of environmental allergens is perennial non-allergic rhinitis (PNAR), sometimes called vasomotor rhinitis. PNAR patients most often will complain of irritants (such as cigarette smoke, perfumes, scented candles, air fresheners, household cleaning agents, and sometimes flower scents such as rose and lily) that cause nasal symptoms. Although some respond to the usual rhinitis medications, most will respond best to Astelin®, an antihistamine nasal spray that, ironically, works well on non-allergic rhinitis. Astelin® works because most of these PNAR cases are due to histamine released from mast cells secondary to non-IgE-mediated processes such as estrogen binding to its receptor-α on mast cells (discussed at length in previous sections). Patients who present with allergy symptoms but who have negative skin tests, and in addition have comorbidities suggestive of hormone imbalance syndrome, should be evaluated for hormone imbalance and have the imbalance corrected; this will usually help the patients not only with their allergies but the other estrogen-related comorbidities. While measuring the hormones, do not forget to include vitamin D in the basic hormone panel. (Vitamin D deficiency is rampant and is associated not only with heart disease but also with allergic diseases such as asthma and perhaps allergic rhinitis.)

Allergic diseases are on the rise, and recent allergy literature indicates that adult-onset allergies are more prevalent in women and the obese. Obesity is highly associated with estrogen dominance; women with increased estrogen dominance due to endogenous (own production) estrogens (estradiol, estrone, and estriol) coupled with xenoestrogens (environmental estrogens) and phytoestrogens (plant-based estrogens), tend to have the highest rate of adult-onset allergic diseases, as demonstrated in Chapter 1. In all cases of rhinitis, sinusitis, and conjunctivitis, prime-age women, ages 18-44, had the highest rates. More information about the estrogen epidemic and obesity and related comorbidities can be found in my book *Hormone Imbalance Syndrome: America's Silent Plague — Uncovering the Roots of the Obesity Epidemic and Common Diseases*.

To find out what causes nasal symptoms, eczema, and asthma symptoms, skin testing is performed. Chapter 4 presents the rationale for skin testing and AIT.

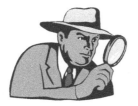

SKIN TESTING AND ALLERGY VACCINE

Two reasons for performing skin testing are:

1. Timing of medication treatment
- Spring symptoms are due to tree pollens
- Summer symptoms are due to grass pollens
- Fall symptoms are due to weed pollens
- Year-round (perennial) symptoms are due to cat, dog, dust mites, molds, cockroach, horse, rabbit, guinea pig, hamster, gerbil, mouse, rat, etc.

Patients with spring or fall allergies should pre-empt their season by starting the medication therapy two weeks prior to the beginning of the season, instead of just reacting to the symptoms. Patients with year-round allergies should treat symptoms year-round.

2. Allergy vaccine
Allergy medications are only palliative and will not provide a long-term resolution of the allergy symptoms. The allergy

vaccine is conceived for long-term relief from allergens. The following will provide an in-depth discussion of allergen sensitization, immunotherapy, and immune cells' response to the various forms of allergy vaccine.

Allergic rhinitis is an important clinical problem, as it affects 20%-40% of the U.S. population. Allergies to various pollens (e.g., trees, grasses, weeds) characteristically result in seasonal rhinitis symptoms, commonly termed "hay fever," whereas sensitivity to certain perennial aeroallergens such as dust mites, molds, cockroaches, and animals (cats, dogs, mice, rats, rabbits, hamsters, horses) results in chronic/perennial/year-round allergic rhinitis. A subset of patients with persistent allergic rhinitis suffers with the sequel of chronic sinusitis.

The medical management of allergic rhinitis, allergic asthma, and allergic sinusitis includes allergen avoidance, pharmacotherapy, and immunotherapy. Immunotherapy is generally considered to be appropriate for patients in whom "hay fever" symptoms cannot be adequately controlled by environmental control and pharmacotherapy, or in whom compliance with daily maintenance medications is a problem, or in whom medications have caused adverse events.

Patients suspected of having an allergic component to their rhinitis, asthma, or sinusitis are also tested for allergies, and if the test is positive, they are started on pharmacotherapy alone as indicated by NHLBI or GINA guidelines, or started on immunotherapy in addition to standard rhinitis, asthma, or sinusitis therapy. Studies have shown that this type of adjuvant immunotherapy, as well as dosage reduction of the standard therapy in children older than 5 and in adults, helps to reduce rhinitis, asthma, and sinusitis symptoms. Although efficacy studies and side-effect profiles of immunotherapy in this setting exist, no studies have investigated the sensitization patterns over time, the rate of asthma development and health care utilization, and cost-effectiveness when immunotherapy is used as adjuvant to standard therapy in the treatment of mild asthma, rhinitis, or sinusitis in mono-allergen-sensitized children up to age 5 (18 months to 5 years), compared with standard therapy alone.

Two European studies (Di Rienzo, et al., *Clinical Experimental Allergy*, 2005 and Fiocchi, et al., *Annals of Allergy, Asthma and Immunology*, 2005) have looked at sublingual immunotherapy (SLIT) — allergen extracts formulated for drops under the tongue — in children younger than 5 years. The first study (Di Rienzo, et al.) enrolled children aged 3-5 years with respiratory allergy receiving SLIT, and they were followed up for at least two years. A diary card for side effects was filled out by parents at each dose given. Local and systemic side effects were graded as mild (no intervention, no dose adjustment), moderate (medical treatment and/or dose reduction), or severe (life-threatening/hospitalization/emergency care). The comparative safety of different allergens and regimens was also assessed.

One hundred and twenty-six children (mean age 4.2 years, 67 male) were included. Seventy-six (60%) had rhinitis with asthma, 34 (27%) had rhinitis only, and 16 (13%) had only asthma.

Immunotherapy was prescribed for mites (62% of the children), grasses (22.2%), Parietaria (11.9%), Alternaria (2.4%), and olive

(1.5%). Eighteen children underwent an accelerated build-up. The total number of doses was about 39,000. Nine side effects were reported in seven children (5.6% patients and 0.2/1000 doses). Two episodes of oral itching and one of abdominal pain were mild. Six gastrointestinal side effects were controlled by reducing the dose. All side effects occurred during up-dosing phase. No difference in terms of safety among the allergens used was observed.

The study concluded that SLIT is safe also in children under the age of 5 years.

The second study's objective was to assess the safety of high-dose SLIT in a group of children younger than 5 years (Fiocchi et al., *Annals of Allergy, Asthma and Immunology*, 2005).

Methods: Sixty-five children (51 boys and 14 girls; age range 38-80 months; mean ± SD age 60 ± 10 years; median age 60 months) were included in this observational study. They were treated with SLIT with a build-up phase of 11 days, culminating in a top dose of 300 IR (Index of Reactivity) and a maintenance phase of 300 IR three times a week. The allergens used were house dust mites in 42 patients, grass pollen in 11 patients, olive pollen in 5 patients, Parietaria pollen in 4 patients, and cypress pollen in 3 patients. All adverse reactions and changes in the treatment schedule were compared in two subgroups: children 38-60 months old and children 61-80 months old.

Results: The average cumulative dose of SLIT was 36,900 IR. Adverse reactions were observed in 11 children, none of them severe enough to require discontinuation of immunotherapy. Six reactions occurred in the 60-months-or-younger age group, and 7 in the older-than-60-months age group, with no differences between these two groups. The study concluded that high-dose immunotherapy in children younger than 5 years does not cause more adverse reactions than in children aged 5-7 years. There is no reason to forbear studies on safety and efficacy of these preparations in young children.

Another study from the U.K. (Robert et al., *JACI*, 2006) looked at enrolled children (3-16 years) with a history of seasonal allergic asthma sensitized to grass pollen (P pratense) and requiring at least 200 mg of inhaled beclomethasone equivalent per day. Subjects with symptomatic asthma or rhinoconjunctivitis outside the grass pollen season were excluded. The primary outcome measure was a combined asthma symptom-medication score during the second pollen season. Secondary outcome measures included end-point titration skin-prick testing and conjunctival and bronchial provocation testing to allergen, sputum eosinophilia, exhaled nitric oxide, and adverse events. Thirty-nine subjects were enrolled. Thirty-five subjects provided data for analysis. All patients were pretreated with loratidine and topical anesthetic creams, and subjects were observed for 60 minutes after each injection. Standard guidelines were used in the case of intercurrent illness or adverse reactions.

The use of SIT (specific immunotherapy, or allergy shots) was associated with a substantial reduction in asthma symptom-medication score compared with that after placebo ($P < .04$). There were also significant reductions in cutaneous ($P < .002$), conjunctival ($P < .02$), and bronchial ($P < .01$) reactivity to allergen after SIT compared with that after placebo. The two groups had similar levels of airway inflammation, despite a trend toward less inhaled steroid use in the active group. No serious adverse events were reported, and no subjects withdrew because of adverse events. The study concluded that SIT is effective and well-tolerated in children with seasonal allergic asthma to grass (see references in the bibliographical notes of Chapter 4). To understand the effect of allergen immunotherapy, allergen sensitization and allergic reaction are described in the next section.

Allergen Sensitization, Allergic Reaction, and Treatment

Allergen **s**ensitization and reaction cascade are depicted in the diagram below.

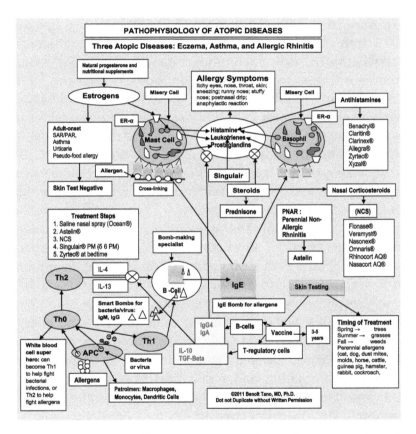

I am reiterating the allergen sensitization and reaction cascade information from Chapter 2 in this paragraph as a reminder.

In this diagram, start in the bottom left with the APC's, antigen-presenting cells: macrophages, monocytes, dendritic cells, and sometimes B cells, that I earlier called the patrolmen of the body. These cells pick up a bacteria/virus, other infectious pathogens, and allergens and present them to the "white blood cell super hero": the Th0 cell. The Th0 cell, in presence of allergens, converts to Th2 cells. The first natural exposure to the allergen leads Th2 cells to produce IL-4 and IL-13 (remember that interleukins 4 and 13 are chemicals used by the Th2 cells to communicate with the B cells), which stimulate B cells to produce IgE antibodies (view the IgE as a smart bomb for allergens). The IgE antibodies bind to their receptors on the mast cells and basophils. Upon re-exposure to the same allergen, the allergen binds and cross-links the IgE antibodies on the surface of the mast cells and basophils. The cross-linking of the IgE antibodies leads to degranulation of the mast cells and basophils with mediator release (histamine, leukotrienes, and prostaglandins — see complete list in Table 20). Medication therapy (antihistamines, leukotriene receptor antagonists, nasal corticosteroids, and occasionally, prednisone) targets these mediators. The Th2 cells, in addition to IL-4 and IL-13, also produce IL-5, which generates a late-phase response by stimulating eosinophils (white blood cells specialized in killing parasites but that contribute to allergic inflammation) to produce toxic proteins (major basic protein, or MBP, and eosinophilic cationic protein, ECP, involved in chronic inflammation and tissue destruction), leukotrienes, IL-3, and IL-6 (IL-6 is also involved in chronic inflammation). Basophils are also stimulated to produce mediators and IL-4 (see Table 20 for complete list).

All the medications are palliative and will not eliminate the symptoms for a long period of time. Skin testing is therefore performed to guide timing of the medication therapy and for deciding on allergen immunotherapy (AIT), also known as allergy vaccine. The vaccine stimulates T-regulatory cells to produce IL-10 and TGF-beta, and also stimulates the B cells to produce IgG4 and IgA instead of IgE. These four "good chemicals" block IL-4 and IL-13 release from the Th2 cells and therefore block the communication line between the Th2 cells and the B cells, which prevents IgE release from the B cells. These good chemicals also block the mediator released from mast cells and basophils. Over time, if the T-regulatory cells and the B cells are trained long enough to recognize the allergens (it usually takes about three to five years for full recognition), they will do the job on their own, and no allergic reactions will occur for a very long period of time.

If, after two to three years, a person is not doing well on the immunotherapy, he should be retested and the AIT protocol adjusted. Whether a patient outgrows his allergies or not depends on the strength of the AIT extracts. Low-dose therapy is not likely to stimulate the T-regulatory cells and the B cells to quickly recognize the antigens. Too high a dose may cause anaphylactic reactions. Hence, immunotherapy is an art and should be formulated judiciously for an optimal result. I am of the opinion that patients should be retested by year three to see if they have outgrown any of their allergens, and to reformulate the AIT protocol to take into account the sensitization pattern at year three, so as to clear all symptoms by year five. Occasionally, patients have outgrown their allergens by year three or five, but they still have nasal symptoms. In this situation, chemical sensitivity or estrogens are the culprits. Recall that in most cases of adult-onset allergies, the major inciting factor is estrogen-induced mast cell and basophil degranulation. Although the medication therapy (antihistamines, LTRA, nasal corticosteroids) in estrogen-induced mast cell mediator release is the same as pollen-induced mediator release, these patients may also benefit from bioidentical hormone (hormone with the same structure as the one produced in the body) therapy.

TABLE 20

MAST CELL AND BASOPHIL MEDIATORS

PRODUCTS OF MAST CELL ACTIVATION	PRODUCTS OF BASOPHIL ACTIVATION
Histamine	Histamine
PROTEASES	**PROTEASES**
-Tryptase	-Tryptase
-Carboxypeptidase	-Elastase
-Chymase	-Cathepsin G
-Cathepsin G	
-Elastase	
-Plasminogen Activator	
-Renin	
-Matrix Metalloprotease 9	
PROTEOGLYCANS	**PROTEOGLYCANS**
-Heparin	-Heparin
-Chodroitin sulfate	-Chodroitin sulfate
CYTOKINES	**CYTOKINES**
-IL-4, IL-5, IL-6, IL-8, IL-13, GM-CSF, TNF-α	-IL-4, IL-8, IL-13, MIP-1α
-Fibroblast growth factor, stem cell factor	-IgE-dependent histamine-releasing factor
LIPID MEDIATORS	**LIPID MEDIATORS**
-Prostaglandin D2	
-Leukotriene C4	-Leukotriene C4
-Platelet-Activating Factor	-Platelet-Activating Factor
OTHER ENZYMES	**OTHER ENZYMES**
-β-hexosaminidase	-β-hexosaminidase
-B-Glucuronidase	**BASIC PROTEINS**
-Arylsulfatase	-Basogranulin, 2D7 antigen
	-Eosinophil major basic protein
	-Eosinophil cationic protein
	-Eosinophil-derived neurotoxin

Table 20 presents: Mast cell with its activation products and basophil with its activation products.

Adapted from JACI, vol. 120, issue 1, supplement, pp S2-S24, July 2007

Summary of the Effects of Allergen Immunotherapy

Allergen SIT is associated with:

- decrease in IL-4 and IL-5 production by CD4+ T cells
- a shift from Th2 cytokine pattern toward increased interferon-γ (IFN)-γ production
- a rise in allergen-blocking IgG antibodies, particularly of the IgG4 class, which supposedly block allergen and IgE-facilitated antigen presentation
- generation of IgE modulating CD8+ T cell and reduction in the number of mast cells and eosinophils, including the release of mediators

Induction of a tolerant state in peripheral T cells represents an essential step in allergen immunotherapy. Peripheral T-cell tolerance is characterized mainly by suppressed proliferative and cytokine responses against the major allergens and T-cell recognition sites. The T-cell tolerance is initiated by autocrine action of IL-10, which is increasingly produced by the antigen-specific T cells.

Tolerized T cells can be reactivated to produce either of the distinct Th1 or Th2 cytokine patterns depending on the cytokine present in the tissue microenvironment, and thus direct allergen immunotherapy toward successful or unsuccessful treatment.

The response to allergen immunotherapy is mostly mediated by T-regulatory cells and B cells.

Effects of T-Regulatory Cell Cytokines

The IL-10 and TGF-β (TGF-Beta) released by the T-regulatory cells:

- decrease the IgE production by the B cells and increase their production of IgA and IgG4
- decrease the IgE-dependent activation of mast cells and basophils
- decrease survival and activation of eosinophils
- suppress mucus production by the epithelial cells and reduce airway hyper-reactivity
- decrease the antigen presentation capacity of dendritic cells
- decrease Th2 cytokines (L-4, IL-13) production and suppression of their proliferation

Immunotherapy is the most cost-effective allergic rhinitis treatment in the long run. However, not everyone qualifies for immunotherapy, and there is the risk of anaphylactic reaction. The allergy societies therefore recommend medication therapy first and if this fails, immunotherapy is then considered. Revisiting our pathophysiology diagram, repeated below to show clarity, it is clear that medication therapy is aimed at blocking the different mediators released by the mast cells and basophils. There have also been attempts at blocking the mediators released by eosinophils. Chapter 5 brings to light the pathophysiology-based medication therapy of allergic disease.

PATHOPHYSIOLOGY OF ATOPIC DISEASES

Three Atopic Diseases: Eczema, Asthma, and Allergic Rhinitis

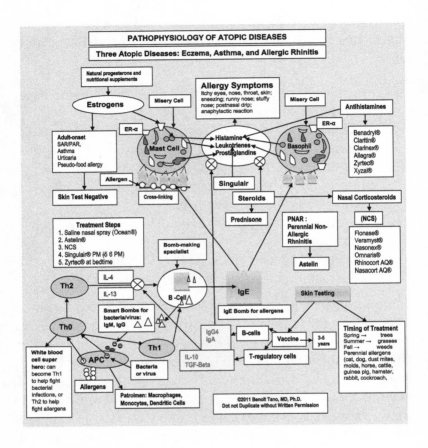

Natural progesterone and nutritional supplements

Estrogens

Misery Cell

Allergy Symptoms
Itchy eyes, nose, throat, skin; sneezing; runny nose; stuffy nose; postnasal drip; anaphylactic reaction

Misery Cell

Antihistamines

ER-α

ER-α

Benadryl®
Claritin®
Clarinex®
Allegra®
Zyrtec®
Xyzal®

Adult-onset
SAR/PAR,
Asthma
Urticaria
Pseudo-food allergy

Mast Cell

Histamine
Leukotrienes
Prostaglandins

Basophil

Allergen

Singulair

Skin Test Negative

Cross-linking

Steroids

Nasal Corticosteroids

Prednisone

PNAR :
Perennial Non-Allergic Rhinitis

(NCS)

Flonase®
Veramyst®
Nasonex®
Omnaris®
Rhinocort AQ®
Nasacort AQ®

Treatment Steps
1. Saline nasal spray (Ocean®)
2. Astelin®
3. NCS
4. Singulair® PM (5 6 PM)
5. Zyrtec® at bedtime

Astelin

Bomb-making specialist

Th2

IL-4

IL-13

B -Cell

IgE

Skin Testing

Smart Bombs for bacteria/virus:
IgM, IgG

IgE Bomb for allergens

Th0

Th1

IgG4
IgA

B-cells

Vaccine

3-5 years

Timing of Treatment
Spring → trees
Summer → grasses
Fall → weeds
Perennial allergens (cat, dog, dust mites, molds, horse, cattle, guinea pig, hamster, rabbit, cockroach,

IL-10
TGF-Beta

T-regulatory cells

White blood cell super hero: can become Th1 to help fight bacterial infections, or Th2 to help fight allergens

APC

Bacteria or virus

Allergens

Patroimen: Macrophages, Monocytes, Dendritic Cells

©2011 Benoit Tano, MD, Ph.D.
Dot not Duplicate without Written Permission

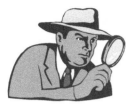

MEDICATION THERAPY AND TREATMENT TECHNIQUES

Treatment success of allergic rhinitis is based on the pathophysiology of this disease. In my one-hour visits with patients, I take a thorough history and perform a physical examination. After the history and physical examination, I discuss the pathophysiology of atopic (allergic) diseases as depicted above. The pathophysiology of atopic diseases diagram shows the interactions between the white blood cells that lead to the release of toxic mediators from the misery cells (mast cells and basophils). I then explain how to block each of these toxic mediators (antihistamines to block histamine, leukotriene receptor antagonists to block leukotrienes, and NCS's to block all of the mediators). Finally, I explain perennial non-allergic rhinitis (PNAR), often called vasomotor rhinitis or chemical sensitivity.

Eighty-five percent of patients with allergy symptoms also have PNAR. All smokers with allergy symptoms also have this condition. Smokers will indicate that cigarette smoke does not bother them. However, once they quit smoking, most smokers cannot tolerate the smell of cigarette smoke. PNAR patients benefit from antihistamine nasal sprays such as Astelin® or Patanase®. Medication therapy, in general, is a palliative and does not cure allergies. The more permanent solution for allergic rhinitis is to desensitize patients with allergen immuno-therapy protocol. Desensitization is the principal reason for skin testing. If a patient has seasonal allergies, he does not have to take medication year-round. He can start taking his medications two weeks prior to the start of the season. I usually explain the association of the different allergens with their season. I explain how desensitization works by revealing the role of T-regulatory cells and B cells in this process. Once the pathophysiology is explained, I then teach the patient how to use the different medications as described below:

Start with Ocean® Nasal Spray

There are many saline nasal sprays and nasal washes in the market. However, they are not all created equal. If you pay attention to the descriptions of these saline nasal sprays, many report that they compare to Ocean® nasal spray. This means that Ocean® is the standard and all others are mimics. I have tried many of these saline nasal sprays myself and found that Ocean® works better. I therefore recommend that my patients use Ocean® nasal spray not only as a moisturizer for the nose but also for control of postnasal drip. The persistent, annoying, often embarrassing postnasal drip that causes most allergy sufferers to clear their throats all the time responds well to Ocean® nasal spray. However, you have to do it right for good results. How do you administer Ocean® nasal spray for better results? I have to call this one Dr. Tano's Technique to claim fame to something.

1. Keep one Ocean® nasal spray bottle in the shower and one with you at all times.

2. While in a hot shower, with nice steam, tilt your head back and gently press the Ocean® nasal spray bottle to let the saline drip slowly into both nostrils, making sure that all the nasal membranes are moisturized. Deliver a generous amount of the nasal spray solution into both nostrils until you get plenty in the throat. Make sure the quantity in the throat is large enough to gargle with. Then, cough it up and blow the nose.

    Repeat this process five times while in the shower, and clean the nose with water afterward. If you have a stuffy nose, use the nasal spray several times until you can breathe through the nose. Throughout the day, use the spray three times or more for better results.

3. Use Ocean® nasal spray to prevent colds. When you have a sore throat, what do most people tell you to do for relief? Most folks will recommend gargling with hot salt water. Ocean® nasal spray is better salt water, since it is made isotonic to the secretions from the nose. Using my technique described above, you may prevent getting colds for seven days. As soon as you feel cold symptoms, start using your Ocean® nasal spray as described above. If you are diligent about it, your cold will not last more than two days. I even tell my patients to start using Ocean® nasal spray soon after exposure to someone with a cold to avoid catching the cold.

4. Use Ocean® nasal spray to prevent recurrent sinus infections. Sinus infections occur when mucus accumulates in the sinuses and becomes a breeding ground

for bacteria. By draining the sinuses regularly, sinus infections will not occur. If you use Ocean® nasal spray as instructed above, you may be able to drain your sinuses and hence avoid recurrent sinus infections. If, after using the nasal spray you continue to have these symptoms, you should see your allergist for a CT scan of the sinuses for evaluation of chronic sinusitis that may respond to a long-term antibiotic therapy (usually four to six weeks of antibiotic therapy is needed to treat chronic sinusitis effectively). If you start on a long course of antibiotics for your sinusitis, make sure you eat yogurt or take probiotics to prevent a disruption to intestinal flora.

Ocean® nasal spray is one of the cheapest ways of treating some allergy symptoms. The 3.5-oz (104 ml) dose costs about $4.00 in some stores.

NCS and Antihistamine Nasal Spray Techniques that Work

- The technique for using nasal corticosteroids (NCS's) such as Flonase®, Veramyst®, Nasonex®, Omnaris®, Rhinocort AQ®, or Nasacort®, and antihistamine nasal sprays such as Astelin® and Patanase®, is the same for all these nasal spray medications and differs from the Ocean® nasal spray technique.

Make sure to wait about 10 minutes after using Ocean® nasal spray before using any of the other nasal sprays. If the nose is clean, there will be less sneezing and less runny nose after using the steroid or antihistamine nasal sprays. If you blow the nose after using these medications, you will not get the full benefit.

* To use any of the NCS or antihistamine nasal sprays:

1. Bend the head slightly forward.
2. Insert the nozzle of the bottle into the left nostril as far as possible, slightly point the nozzle toward the left eye, and deliver two sprays. Lift the head up and pinch the nose gently for the spray to cover the nasal membranes.
3. Repeat the same process for the right nostril, making sure the nozzle of the bottle points toward the right eye. (Pointing the nozzle toward the   eyes   prevents spraying on the nasal septum. Spraying on the septum leads to nosebleeds, stinging and burning experienced by many patients.)
4. Most of all **do not** sniff during the spray or after spraying. Sniffing causes the spray to be lost into the throat and, for some patients, irritation from the NCS may even cause a sore throat. If you sniff your nasal spray, you will be wasting your time, your money, and you will not get the expected relief.

NOTE: Astelin® tastes bitter and if you make a mistake and sniff it during or after the spray in the nose, you will taste it in your throat and mouth. You may gargle with water to relieve the bitter taste.

Sequence of Nasal Sprays

If you have concomitant seasonal/perennial allergic rhinitis and PNAR, you may need a combination therapy for better relief from your symptoms.

The most optimal combination is:

1. Ocean® nasal spray
2. Astelin®
3. A NCS
4. Singulair®
5. Zyrtec®

Start with Ocean® nasal spray, wait about 5-10 minutes, and then use the Astelin®. Wait another 5-10 minutes and then use the NCS (Veramyst®, Nasonex®, Omnaris®, Rhinocort AQ®, or Nasacort AQ®). For most rhinitis sufferers, the adequate amount of Astelin® or NCS is 2 x 2 x 2 (which means two sprays in each nostril twice a day). Most of the time, the 2 x 2 x 1 or the 1 x 2 x 1 recommended by most health care providers does not do the job. Once acute exacerbation of the rhinitis symptoms improves, then use 2 x 2 x 1. In children, use 1 x 2 x 1 if nasal symptoms are mild. For severe nasal symptoms in children, a short course of using the NCS 2 x 2 x 1 is optimal; then switch to 1 x 2 x 1 when symptoms improve.

For the very young (age 1) with severe nasal symptoms, Nasonex®, which is approved for age 2 and above, can be used off-label (even though not approved for ages below 2). In this case, use Nasonex® 1 x 2 x 1.

For patients with PNAR, using Flonase®, which has a light floral scent, may not be optimal; these patients will not tolerate the scent, and they will do better with any of the other NCS's.

PNAR sufferers beware! Some insurance plans will refuse to cover other NCS's and direct everyone to Flonase®, which may not be optimal or cost-effective for both patients and insurance companies. In this case, you may want to ask your health care provider to obtain a prior authorization for another brand of NCS.

Take the Singulair® around supper time (5:00-6:00 p.m.) because the leukotrienes are released at night, and taking the Singulair® in the morning will defeat the purpose. Taking it at bedtime (around 9:00-10:00 p.m. for most people) is too late.

Finally, take your Zyrtec® at bedtime. Children 6 years and older can take Zyrtec® 10 mg.

Zyrtec® syrup does not seem to do the job as well, and many children 2 to 5 years old will do better with chewable Zyrtec® 5 mg tablets.

Allergic Conjunctivitis Treatment

For allergic conjunctivitis, you may use an over-the-counter eye drop such as Zaditor® or prescription eye drops such as Patanol®, Elestat®, or Pataday®. If you use prescription eye drops, do not expect results immediately. These medications have an antihistamine and a mast cell stabilizer. It takes about two weeks for mast cell stabilization, so be patient.

In addition to these nasal medications and eye drops, I often recommend orthomolecular therapy.

Orthomolecular Therapy

"Orthomolecular medicine, as conceptualized by double-Nobel laureate Linus Pauling, aims to restore the optimum environment of the body by correcting imbalances or deficiencies based on individual biochemistry, using substances natural to the body such as vitamins, minerals, amino acids, trace elements and fatty acids." The term "orthomolecular" was first used by Linus Pauling in a paper he wrote in the journal *Science* in 1968. The key idea in orthomolecular medicine is that genetic factors affect not only the physical characteristics of individuals, but also their biochemical milieu. Biochemical pathways of the body have significant genetic variability, and diseases such as atherosclerosis, cancer, schizophrenia, and depression are associated with specific biochemical abnormalities which are causal or contributing factors of the illness (definition from www.orthomed.org).

Through anti-aging fellowship training programs, many health care providers are now learning the principles of orthomolecular medicine to better help their patients.

Biomonitoring, as reported by the CDC, has found harmful chemicals in human blood and urine, and many of these chemicals have been shown by scientific studies to increase estrogen, decrease thyroid function, and decrease androgens (male hormones produced by both men and women). These chemicals are now known as endocrine-disrupting chemicals (EDC's). EDC's not only cause a great deal of the obesity epidemic (and obviously the obesity comorbidities such as diabetes, hypertension, hyperlipidemia, hypothyroidism), but also the growing allergy epidemic (which is estrogen-driven until proven otherwise), and the myriad of other symptoms treated by health care professionals.

How do you protect yourself and your family against pollution and this epidemic of internal chemical disruption? Orthomolecular therapy may contribute to your overall well-being.

Orthomolecular Approach to Allergic Rhinitis

I recommend that my adult patients with rhinitis symptoms take antioxidants, vitamin D, and minerals. I usually recommend:

- B-complex vitamins
- Buffered vitamin C
- Co-enzyme Q10
- Vitamin E (make sure to use mixed tocopherols)
- Omega-3 fish oil (EPA/DHA)
- L-carnitine
- Astaxanthin
- Vitamin D and multiminerals such as calcium, magnesium, potassium, zinc, manganese, iron, boron, iodine, chromium, selenium, vanadium, and molybdenum
- Broad-spectrum digestive enzymes and probiotics supplementation

Some nutritional supplements may interact with your other prescribed medications, and you should therefore consult with your health care provider prior to embarking on these supplements.

Supplementation with antioxidants such as vitamins C and L-carnitine has been growing rapidly in the past few years as research on harmful free radicals intensifies. Free radicals are atoms, ions, or molecules with one or more unpaired electrons that bind to and destroy cellular compounds. Dietary antioxidants disarm free radicals through a number of different mechanisms. Foremost, they bind to the free electrons, "pairing up" with them, creating an innocuous cellular compound that the body can eliminate as waste. Recent research suggests that a synergistic combination of antioxidants is more effective than the total effect of each antioxidant taken alone.

The benefit of antioxidants, minerals, and vitamin D go beyond oxidation and encompass better blood pressure, glucose and lipid controls, and better control of allergic diseases.

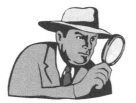

OVERALL
SUMMARY

- Atopic diseases are on the rise.
- Many patients are treated by their primary care health providers, who have difficulty controlling the symptoms because of lack of understanding of the pathophysiology of atopic diseases. This guide has shed some light on the pathophysiology of the atopic diseases and shown how a combination therapy is often required to treat the coexisting atopic diseases such as allergic rhinitis and asthma, and non-allergic rhinitis that is present concomitantly in about 85% of allergic rhinitis sufferers. Combination therapy is optimal to shorten the duration of a rhinitis exacerbation.
- Many allergy patients do not understand what is causing their allergy symptoms and therefore do not take their medications as they should. When they see their health care providers, they also get medications that do not work. Lower-end antihistamines such as Benadryl® and Claritin® are tried first by many, whereas more potent antihistamines such as Zyrtec® and Allegra® are over-the-counter. When NCS's are

prescribed, often the patient is not shown how to use these nasal sprays and therefore many end up with nosebleeds or sore throats that lead the patients to discontinue these NCS's which, when used correctly, are very effective in controlling the rhinitis symptoms.

- Adult-onset allergies are on the rise and in most cases are due to estrogen dominance. There is an estrogen epidemic in America and the world today that is directly related to pesticides/herbicides sprayed in farmlands and chemicals used in the house. These pesticides, household cleaning agents, cosmetics, and cosmeceuticals have three major effects: they increase estrogen, decrease thyroid function, and decrease androgens. These three effects lead to obesity and its comorbidities. Increased estrogen is an independent risk factor for adult-onset rhinitis symptoms. As reported in Chapter 4, when the endogenous estrogens, xenoestrogens, and phytoestrogens bind to the estrogen receptor-alpha (ER-alpha) on mast cells, they cause mast cell degranulation just like pollens and other environmental allergens do. Women who have a large initial endowment of endogenous estrogens (estradiol, estrone, and estriol) tend to bear the highest atopic disease burden. Women also bear the highest burden for obesity and its comorbidities. A complete analysis of the contributions of agrichemicals, household chemicals, cosmetics, and cosmeceuticals to obesity and its comorbidities can be found in my book *Hormone Imbalance Syndrome: America's Silent Plague — Uncovering the Roots of the Obesity Epidemic and Common Diseases.*

- The next Allergy Detective episode will uncover the roots of the growing food allergy epidemic.

APPENDIX A

TABLE 1

Patient and hospital characteristics for ICD-9-CM first-listed diagnosis code 477.0 Rhinitis Due to Pollen

	All ED visits (those that resulted in admission to the hospital and those that did not)	Only hospital visits that originated in the ED	Only ED visits that ended in discharge (no hospital admission)	Standard errors		
				All ED Visits	Admitted to the hospital from the ED	Discharged from the ED
All discharges	7,067 (100.00%)	*	7,027 (100.00%)	703	*	702
Age (mean)	27.42	43.62	27.32	0.75	0.75	0.75
Age group <1	153 (2.16%)		153 (100.00%)	44		44 (0.00%)
1-17	2,364 (33.45%)	*	2,355 (99.64%)	297	*	297 (0.26%)
18-44	3,179 (44.98%)	*	3,167 (99.64%)	347	*	346 (0.21%)
45-64	1,098 (15.53%)	*	1,090 (99.31%)	123	*	123 (0.51%)
65-84	257 (3.63%)	*	243 (94.85%)	40	*	39 (2.95%)
85+	*		*	*		*
Sex Male	3,076 (43.53%)	*	3,059 (99.46%)	316	*	315 (0.27%)
Female	3,991 (56.47%)	*	3,967 (99.40%)	414	*	414 (0.28%)
Median income for zipcode Low	2,425 (34.32%)	*	2,408 (99.29%)	323	*	322 (0.45%)
Not low	4,493 (63.58%)	*	4,480 (99.70%)	508	*	507 (0.17%)
Missing	149 (2.10%)	*	139 (93.24%)	33	*	32 (4.73%)
Region Northeast	2,039 (28.86%)	*	2,021 (99.07%)	411	*	411 (0.50%)
Midwest	1,177 (16.65%)	*	1,172 (99.59%)	189	*	187 (0.38%)
South	2,391 (33.84%)	*	2,374 (99.29%)	314	*	312 (0.44%)
West	1,460 (20.66%)		1,460 (100.00%)	438		438 (0.00%)

* Denotes missing values   HCUP-2008

Allergic rhinitis due to pollen is more prevalent in women at 56.5%, and is seen more in the prime-age group (ages 18-44) at 45%, followed by the young (ages 1-17) at 33.5%, and then older adults (ages 45-64) at 15.5%, and finally ages 65-84 at 3.6%. Pollen allergy is more prevalent in the South at 33.8%, followed by the Northeast at 28.9%, the West at 20.7%, and finally the Midwest at 16.7%.

TABLE 2

Patient and hospital characteristics for ICD-9-CM first-listed diagnosis code 477.8 Allergic Rhinitis Nec (not elsewhere classified)

		All ED visits (those that resulted in admission to the hospital and those that did not)	Only hospital visits that originated in the ED	Only ED visits that ended in discharge (no hospital admission)	Standard errors		
					All ED Visits	Admitted to the hospital from the ED	Discharged from the ED
All discharges		3,971 (100.00%)	*	3,941 (100.00%)	243	*	242
Age (mean)		29.59	29.56	29.59	0.74	0.74	0.74
Age group	<1	*		*	*	*	*
	1-17	1,216 (30.63%)	*	1,211 (99.55%)	106	*	106 (0.45%)
	18-44	1,847 (46.51%)	*	1,831 (99.15%)	128	*	128 (0.43%)
	45-64	648 (16.31%)	*	639 (98.72%)	74	*	74 (0.92%)
	65-84	219 (5.51%)		219 (100.00%)	32		32 (0.00%)
	85+	*		*	*		*
Sex	Male	1,490 (37.53%)	*	1,475 (98.95%)	114	*	114 (0.54%)
	Female	2,480 (62.47%)	*	2,467 (99.45%)	164	*	163 (0.32%)
Median income for zipcode	Low	1,361 (34.26%)	*	1,352 (99.34%)	133	*	133 (0.47%)
	Not low	2,501 (62.99%)	*	2,486 (99.40%)	178	*	178 (0.30%)
	Missing	109 (2.75%)	*	104 (95.04%)	27	*	26 (4.87%)
Region	Northeast	911 (22.95%)	*	897 (98.39%)	133	*	133 (1.20%)
	Midwest	842 (21.20%)		842 (100.00%)	124		124 (0.00%)
	South	1,556 (39.20%)	*	1,542 (99.05%)	139	*	138 (0.46%)
	West	661 (16.65%)		661 (100.00%)	80		80 (0.00%)

*Denotes missing values   HCUP-2008

Allergic rhinitis Nec (not elsewhere classified, such as due to pollen) is more prevalent in females at 62.5%, and is seen more in the prime-age group (ages 18-44) at 46.5%, followed by the young (ages 1-17) at 30.6%, older adults (ages 45-64) at 16.3%, and then in ages 65-84 at 5.5%. The South leads with 39.2%, followed by the Northeast at 23%, the Midwest at 21.2%, and the West at 16.7%.

TABLE 3

Patient and hospital characteristics for ICD-9-CM first-listed diagnosis code 477.9 Allergic Rhinitis Nos (not otherwise specified)

		All ED visits (those that resulted in admission to the hospital and those that did not)	Only hospital visits that originated in the ED	Only ED visits that ended in discharge (no hospital admission)	Standard errors		
					All ED Visits	Admitted to the hospital from the ED	Discharged from the ED
All discharges		74,898 (100.00%)	159 (100.00%)	74,739 (100.00%)	3,814	33	3,812
Age (mean)		26.58	53.41	26.52	0.52	0.52	0.52
Age group	<1	2,343 (3.13%)		2,343 (100.00%)	179		179 (0.00%)
	1-17	27,083 (36.16%)	*	27,072 (99.96%)	1,814	*	1,814 (0.02%)
	18-44	30,824 (41.15%)	*	30,786 (99.88%)	1,651	*	1,651 (0.05%)
	45-64	10,800 (14.42%)	65 (0.61%)	10,735 (99.39%)	803	19 (0.18%)	803 (0.18%)
	65-84	3,549 (4.74%)	*	3,507 (98.82%)	227	*	226 (0.36%)
	85+	299 (0.40%)	*	296 (99.00%)	39	*	39 (1.00%)
Sex	Male	33,163 (44.28%)	75 (0.23%)	33,088 (99.77%)	1,713	20 (0.06%)	1,711 (0.06%)
	Female	41,730 (55.72%)	84 (0.20%)	41,646 (99.80%)	2,177	23 (0.06%)	2,177 (0.06%)
	Missing	*		*	*		*
Median income for zipcode	Low	30,119 (40.21%)	*	30,056 (99.79%)	2,346	*	2,346 (0.08%)
	Not low	43,152 (57.61%)	86 (0.20%)	43,065 (99.80%)	2,201	22 (0.05%)	2,199 (0.05%)
	Missing	1,627 (2.17%)	*	1,618 (99.42%)	142	*	141 (0.57%)
Region	Northeast	17,690 (23.62%)	*	17,644 (99.74%)	2,778	*	2,779 (0.12%)
	Midwest	15,742 (21.02%)	*	15,720 (99.86%)	1,550	*	1,549 (0.08%)
	South	31,556 (42.13%)	*	31,482 (99.76%)	1,871	*	1,869 (0.07%)
	West	9,910 (13.23%)	*	9,893 (99.83%)	960	*	959 (0.09%)

*Denotes missing values   HCUP-2008

Allergic rhinitis Nos (not otherwise specified) is more prevalent in females at 55.7%, and is seen more in the prime-age group (ages 18-44) at 41.2%, followed by the young (ages 1-17) at 36.2%, older adults (ages 45-64) at 14.4%, and then ages 65-84 at 4.7%. The South leads at 42.1%, followed by the Northeast at 23.6%, the Midwest at 21%, and the West at 13.2%.

TABLE 4

Patient and hospital characteristics for ICD-9-CM first-listed diagnosis
code 472.0 Chronic Rhinitis

		All ED visits (those that resulted in admission to the hospital and those that did not)	Only hospital visits that originated in the ED	Only ED visits that ended in discharge (no hospital admission)	All ED Visits	Admitted to the hospital from the ED	Discharged from the ED
						Standard errors	
All discharges		19,230 (100.00%)	*	19,173 (100.00%)	2,460	*	2,459
Age (mean)		16.86	49.66	16.76	1.03	1.03	1.03
Age group	<1	4,803 (24.97%)	*	4,790 (99.74%)	726	*	726 (0.16%)
	1-17	7,665 (39.86%)		7,665 (100.00%)	1,296		1,296 (0.00%)
	18-44	3,926 (20.42%)	*	3,916 (99.74%)	348	*	348 (0.15%)
	45-64	1,836 (9.55%)	*	1,825 (99.37%)	188	*	187 (0.37%)
	65-84	816 (4.25%)	*	806 (98.73%)	81	*	80 (0.74%)
	85+	183 (0.95%)	*	171 (93.25%)	31	*	29 (4.76%)
Sex	Male	9,156 (47.61%)	*	9,133 (99.75%)	1,216	*	1,216 (0.13%)
	Female	10,074 (52.39%)	*	10,040 (99.67%)	1,264	*	1,264 (0.12%)
Median income for zipcode	Low	8,267 (42.99%)	*	8,240 (99.67%)	1,443	*	1,442 (0.15%)
	Not low	10,625 (55.25%)	*	10,595 (99.72%)	1,255	*	1,255 (0.12%)
	Missing	338 (1.76%)		338 (100.00%)	57		57 (0.00%)
Region	Northeast	2,022 (10.52%)	*	2,014 (99.59%)	283	*	281 (0.28%)
	Midwest	4,362 (22.68%)	*	4,353 (99.80%)	603	*	601 (0.20%)
	South	11,304 (58.78%)	*	11,269 (99.69%)	2,362	*	2,362 (0.13%)
	West	1,542 (8.02%)	*	1,537 (99.68%)	175	*	175 (0.32%)

*Denotes missing values   HCUP-2008

Chronic rhinitis is more prevalent in females at 52.4%, and is found more in the young (ages 1-17) at 39.9%, followed by children less than one year old at 25%, the prime-aged (ages 18-44) at 20.4%, older adults (ages 45-64) at 9.56%, and finally, ages 65-84 at 4.25%. Chronic rhinitis is more prevalent in the South at 58.8% and the Midwest at 22.7%, followed by the Northeast at 10.5%, and the West at 8%.

TABLE 5

Patient and hospital characteristics for ICD-9-CM first-listed diagnosis code 461.0 Acute Maxillary Sinusitis

		All ED visits (those that resulted in admission to the hospital and those that did not)	Only hospital visits that originated in the ED	Only ED visits that ended in discharge (no hospital admission)	Standard errors		
					All ED Visits	Admitted to the hospital from the ED	Discharged from the ED
All discharges		35,242 (100.00%)	1,707 (100.00%)	33,535 (100.00%)	3,061	112	3,057
Age (mean)		37.58	52.59	36.82	0.33	0.33	0.33
Age group	<1	*	*	*	*	*	*
	1-17	2,851 (8.09%)	121 (4.24%)	2,730 (95.76%)	286	25 (0.91%)	284 (0.91%)
	18-44	21,338 (60.55%)	429 (2.01%)	20,910 (97.99%)	2,064	50 (0.30%)	2,063 (0.30%)
	45-64	8,448 (23.97%)	542 (6.41%)	7,906 (93.59%)	709	63 (0.86%)	703 (0.86%)
	65-84	2,232 (6.33%)	473 (21.17%)	1,759 (78.83%)	167	48 (2.23%)	159 (2.23%)
	85+	322 (0.91%)	124 (38.51%)	198 (61.49%)	41	25 (5.94%)	32 (5.94%)
Sex	Male	12,367 (35.09%)	783 (6.33%)	11,584 (93.67%)	986	69 (0.72%)	983 (0.72%)
	Female	22,871 (64.90%)	923 (4.04%)	21,948 (95.96%)	2,110	82 (0.50%)	2,106 (0.50%)
	Missing	*		*	*		*
Median income for zipcode	Low	11,449 (32.49%)	545 (4.76%)	10,904 (95.24%)	1,341	64 (0.76%)	1,338 (0.76%)
	Not low	23,058 (65.43%)	1,090 (4.73%)	21,968 (95.27%)	2,098	82 (0.53%)	2,093 (0.53%)
	Missing	734 (2.08%)	*	663 (90.27%)	88	*	84 (3.27%)
Region	Northeast	6,799 (19.29%)	358 (5.27%)	6,440 (94.73%)	1,671	51 (1.38%)	1,663 (1.38%)
	Midwest	8,462 (24.01%)	283 (3.34%)	8,179 (96.66%)	1,339	40 (0.72%)	1,341 (0.72%)
	South	16,373 (46.46%)	764 (4.67%)	15,609 (95.33%)	2,147	77 (0.76%)	2,146 (0.76%)
	West	3,609 (10.24%)	302 (8.37%)	3,307 (91.63%)	418	48 (1.59%)	417 (1.59%)

*Denotes missing values   HCUP-2008

Acute maxillary sinusitis is more prevalent in females at 64.9%, and in the prime-age group (ages 18-44) at 60.6%, followed by older adults (ages 45-64) at 24%, the young (ages 1-17) at 8.1%, and finally, in ages 65-84 at 6.33%. Acute maxillary sinusitis is more prevalent in the South at 46.5%, the Midwest at 24%, followed by the Northeast at 19.3%, and the West at 10.2%.

TABLE 6

Patient and hospital characteristics for ICD-9-CM first-listed diagnosis code 473.0 Chronic Maxillary Sinusitis

		All ED visits (those that resulted in admission to the hospital and those that did not)	Only hospital visits that originated in the ED	Only ED visits that ended in discharge (no hospital admission)	Standard errors		
					All ED Visits	Admitted to the hospital from the ED	Discharged from the ED
All discharges		17,573 (100.00%)	1,084 (100.00%)	16,489 (100.00%)	896	79	875
Age (mean)		38.46	47.41	37.87	0.49	0.49	0.49
Age group	<1	*	*	*	*	*	*
	1-17	2,111 (12.01%)	200 (9.46%)	1,912 (90.54%)	223	38 (1.54%)	206 (1.54%)
	18-44	9,334 (53.11%)	237 (2.54%)	9,097 (97.46%)	538	35 (0.39%)	535 (0.39%)
	45-64	4,324 (24.61%)	301 (6.96%)	4,023 (93.04%)	238	38 (0.89%)	233 (0.89%)
	65-84	1,503 (8.55%)	223 (14.83%)	1,280 (85.17%)	105	31 (1.97%)	99 (1.97%)
	85+	268 (1.52%)	100 (37.13%)	168 (62.87%)	40	25 (7.07%)	30 (7.07%)
Sex	Male	6,947 (39.53%)	494 (7.12%)	6,453 (92.88%)	375	52 (0.73%)	363 (0.73%)
	Female	10,622 (60.44%)	590 (5.55%)	10,032 (94.45%)	576	54 (0.52%)	564 (0.52%)
	Missing	*		*	*		*
Median income for zipcode	Low	5,961 (33.92%)	317 (5.31%)	5,644 (94.69%)	502	49 (0.80%)	487 (0.80%)
	Not low	11,120 (63.28%)	727 (6.54%)	10,392 (93.46%)	581	61 (0.56%)	567 (0.56%)
	Missing	493 (2.80%)	*	452 (91.81%)	66	*	63 (3.09%)
Region	Northeast	2,656 (15.12%)	228 (8.59%)	2,428 (91.41%)	400	31 (1.64%)	398 (1.64%)
	Midwest	4,819 (27.42%)	241 (5.00%)	4,578 (95.00%)	441	35 (0.74%)	433 (0.74%)
	South	7,266 (41.35%)	482 (6.63%)	6,784 (93.37%)	600	58 (0.73%)	576 (0.73%)
	West	2,832 (16.12%)	134 (4.72%)	2,698 (95.28%)	295	27 (1.04%)	296 (1.04%)

*Denotes missing values   HCUP-2008

Chronic maxillary sinusitis is more prevalent in females at 60.4%, and is seen more in the prime-age group (ages 18-44) at 53.1%, followed by older adults (ages 45-64) at 24.6%, the young (ages 1-17) at 12.0%, ages 65-84 at 8.6%, and ages 85+ at 1.5%. Chronic maxillary sinusitis is more prevalent in the South at 41.4% and the Midwest at 27.4%, followed by the West at 16.1%, and the Northeast at 15.1%.

TABLE 7

Patient and hospital characteristics for ICD-9-CM first-listed diagnosis code 461.1 Acute Frontal Sinusitis

		All ED visits (those that resulted in admission to the hospital and those that did not)	Only hospital visits that originated in the ED	Only ED visits that ended in discharge (no hospital admission)	Standard errors		
					All ED Visits	Admitted to the hospital from the ED	Discharged from the ED
All discharges		12,716 (100.00%)	249 (100.00%)	12,467 (100.00%)	1,516	37	1,511
Age (mean)		34.96	41.22	34.83	0.42	0.42	0.42
Age group	<1	*		*	*		*
	1-17	1,526 (12.00%)	*	1,501 (98.34%)	203	*	203 (0.73%)
	18-44	7,784 (61.21%)	132 (1.69%)	7,652 (98.31%)	983	25 (0.34%)	978 (0.34%)
	45-64	2,750 (21.63%)	*	2,694 (97.96%)	338	*	337 (0.64%)
	65-84	600 (4.72%)	*	573 (95.45%)	79	*	78 (2.15%)
	85+	*	*	*	*	*	*
Sex	Male	4,698 (36.95%)	110 (2.33%)	4,588 (97.67%)	535	22 (0.52%)	533 (0.52%)
	Female	8,018 (63.05%)	140 (1.74%)	7,878 (98.26%)	1,000	26 (0.36%)	996 (0.36%)
Median income for zipcode	Low	4,661 (36.65%)	56 (1.21%)	4,604 (98.79%)	772	16 (0.38%)	771 (0.38%)
	Not low	7,698 (60.54%)	150 (1.95%)	7,547 (98.05%)	925	26 (0.40%)	924 (0.40%)
	Missing	358 (2.81%)	*	315 (88.13%)	61	*	55 (4.93%)
Region	Northeast	3,056 (24.03%)	*	2,990 (97.85%)	881	*	874 (0.90%)
	Midwest	2,254 (17.72%)	71 (3.14%)	2,183 (96.86%)	481	17 (0.93%)	479 (0.93%)
	South	6,281 (49.40%)	67 (1.06%)	6,214 (98.94%)	1,113	16 (0.30%)	1,112 (0.30%)
	West	1,125 (8.85%)	46 (4.08%)	1,079 (95.92%)	229	14 (1.47%)	230 (1.47%)

*Denotes missing values   HCUP-2008

Acute frontal sinusitis is more prevalent in females at 63.1%, and is seen more in the prime-age group (ages 18-44) at 61.2%, followed by older adults (ages 45-64) at 21.6%, the young (ages 1-17) at 12.0%, and ages 65-84 at 4.7%. Acute frontal sinusitis is more prevalent in the South at 49.4% and the Northeast at 24.0%, followed by the Midwest at 17.7%, and the West at 8.9%.

TABLE 8

Patient and hospital characteristics for ICD-9-CM first-listed diagnosis code 473.1 Chronic Frontal Sinusitis

		All ED visits (those that resulted in admission to the hospital and those that did not)	Only hospital visits that originated in the ED	Only ED visits that ended in discharge (no hospital admission)	Standard errors		
					All ED Visits	Admitted to the hospital from the ED	Discharged from the ED
All discharges		4,085 (100.00%)	169 (100.00%)	3,916 (100.00%)	328	29	326
Age (mean)		35.34	52.46	34.60	0.76	0.76	0.76
Age group	1-17	559 (13.68%)	*	546 (97.68%)	84	*	83 (1.37%)
	18-44	2,380 (58.27%)	54 (2.29%)	2,326 (97.71%)	210	15 (0.63%)	208 (0.63%)
	45-64	816 (19.96%)	*	771 (94.49%)	85	*	83 (1.76%)
	65-84	310 (7.58%)	*	262 (84.51%)	42	*	39 (4.71%)
	85+	*	*	*	*	*	*
Sex	Male	1,777 (43.49%)	95 (5.34%)	1,682 (94.66%)	141	20 (1.13%)	139 (1.13%)
	Female	2,308 (56.51%)	74 (3.22%)	2,234 (96.78%)	217	18 (0.79%)	215 (0.79%)
Median income for zipcode	Low	1,510 (36.96%)	*	1,460 (96.71%)	184	*	182 (1.10%)
	Not low	2,460 (60.21%)	115 (4.67%)	2,345 (95.33%)	205	24 (1.00%)	203 (1.00%)
	Missing	115 (2.83%)	*	111 (95.99%)	30	*	30 (3.99%)
Region	Northeast	788 (19.28%)	*	740 (93.93%)	176	*	176 (2.36%)
	Midwest	981 (24.02%)	*	939 (95.64%)	157	*	156 (1.70%)
	South	1,537 (37.63%)	*	1,497 (97.39%)	192	*	191 (0.91%)
	West	779 (19.07%)	*	741 (95.06%)	124	*	120 (1.50%)

*Denotes missing values   HCUP-2008

Chronic frontal sinusitis is more prevalent in females at 56.5%, and is seen more in the prime-age group (ages 18-44) at 58.3%, followed by older adults (ages 45-64) at 20.0%, the young (ages 1-17) at 13.7%, and ages 65-84 at 7.6%. Chronic frontal sinusitis is more prevalent in the South at 37.6% and the Midwest at 24.0%, followed by the Northeast at 19.3%, and the West at 19.1%.

TABLE 9
Patient and hospital characteristics for ICD-9-CM first-listed diagnosis code 461.2 Acute Ethmoidal Sinusitis

| | | All ED visits (those that resulted in admission to the hospital and those that did not) | Only hospital visits that originated in the ED | Only ED visits that ended in discharge (no hospital admission) | Standard errors | | |
					All ED Visits	Admitted to the hospital from the ED	Discharged from the ED
All discharges		3,372 (100.00%)	573 (100.00%)	2,799 (100.00%)	220	65	211
Age (mean)		39.64	46.46	38.25	0.74	0.74	0.74
Age group	<1	*	*	*	*	*	*
	1-17	429 (12.72%)	94 (21.83%)	335 (78.17%)	53	21 (4.29%)	46 (4.29%)
	18-44	1,593 (47.25%)	160 (10.05%)	1,433 (89.95%)	119	28 (1.76%)	116 (1.76%)
	45-64	904 (26.81%)	143 (15.77%)	761 (84.23%)	85	27 (2.90%)	81 (2.90%)
	65-84	389 (11.53%)	136 (34.96%)	253 (65.04%)	43	39 (8.98%)	44 (8.98%)
	85+	*	*	*	*	*	*
Sex	Male	1,548 (45.92%)	289 (18.65%)	1,260 (81.35%)	122	49 (2.82%)	109 (2.82%)
	Female	1,819 (53.95%)	284 (15.60%)	1,535 (84.40%)	141	39 (2.14%)	135 (2.14%)
	Missing	*		*	*		*
Median income for zipcode	Low	1,039 (30.80%)	182 (17.53%)	857 (82.47%)	111	41 (4.12%)	112 (4.12%)
	Not low	2,206 (65.42%)	366 (16.61%)	1,840 (83.39%)	156	51 (2.10%)	143 (2.10%)
	Missing	127 (3.77%)	*	103 (80.94%)	27	*	25 (7.71%)
Region	Northeast	632 (18.76%)	134 (21.19%)	498 (78.81%)	116	32 (5.11%)	108 (5.11%)
	Midwest	815 (24.18%)	116 (14.22%)	700 (85.78%)	94	26 (2.90%)	86 (2.90%)
	South	1,372 (40.69%)	226 (16.45%)	1,146 (83.55%)	146	35 (2.75%)	142 (2.75%)
	West	552 (16.37%)	*	455 (82.42%)	69	*	72 (6.59%)

*Denotes missing values   HCUP-2008

Acute ethmoidal sinusitis is more prevalent in females at 54.0%, and is seen more in the prime-age group (ages 18-44) at 47.3%, followed by older adults (ages 45-64) at 26.8%, the young (ages 1-17) at 12.7%, and ages 65-84 at 11.5%. Acute ethmoidal sinusitis is more prevalent in the South at 40.7% and the Midwest at 24.2%, followed by the Northeast at 18.8%, and the West at 16.4%.

TABLE 10

Patient and hospital characteristics for ICD-9-CM first-listed diagnosis code 473.2 Chronic Ethmoidal Sinusitis

		All ED visits (those that resulted in admission to the hospital and those that did not)	Only hospital visits that originated in the ED	Only ED visits that ended in discharge (no hospital admission)	Standard errors		
					All ED Visits	Admitted to the hospital from the ED	Discharged from the ED
All discharges		4,969 (100.00%)	485 (100.00%)	4,484 (100.00%)	298	50	285
Age (mean)		39.06	43.32	38.60	0.67	0.67	0.67
Age group	<1	*	*	*	*	*	*
	1-17	675 (13.58%)	104 (15.39%)	571 (84.61%)	70	24 (3.13%)	62 (3.13%)
	18-44	2,409 (48.49%)	121 (5.01%)	2,289 (94.99%)	171	24 (0.98%)	168 (0.98%)
	45-64	1,286 (25.88%)	136 (10.61%)	1,150 (89.39%)	99	23 (1.76%)	95 (1.76%)
	65-84	514 (10.34%)	106 (20.69%)	407 (79.31%)	60	23 (3.79%)	52 (3.79%)
	85+	72 (1.45%)	*	60 (82.98%)	18	*	16 (9.07%)
Sex	Male	2,426 (48.81%)	226 (9.32%)	2,200 (90.68%)	171	31 (1.27%)	166 (1.27%)
	Female	2,539 (51.10%)	259 (10.20%)	2,280 (89.80%)	167	36 (1.33%)	158 (1.33%)
	Missing	*		*	*		
Median income for zipcode	Low	1,512 (30.44%)	164 (10.84%)	1,348 (89.16%)	150	28 (1.87%)	144 (1.87%)
	Not low	3,374 (67.90%)	294 (8.72%)	3,080 (91.28%)	227	41 (1.14%)	217 (1.14%)
	Missing	82 (1.66%)	*	*	24	*	*
Region	Northeast	698 (14.05%)	132 (18.97%)	566 (81.03%)	98	29 (4.20%)	94 (4.20%)
	Midwest	1,237 (24.89%)	86 (6.97%)	1,150 (93.03%)	161	21 (1.63%)	156 (1.63%)
	South	2,364 (47.58%)	211 (8.95%)	2,153 (91.05%)	210	32 (1.23%)	199 (1.23%)
	West	670 (13.49%)	55 (8.18%)	615 (91.82%)	93	15 (2.36%)	92 (2.36%)

*Denotes missing values   HCUP-2008

Chronic ethmoidal sinusitis is more prevalent in females at 51.1%, and is seen more in the prime-age group (ages 18-44) at 48.5%, followed by older adults (ages 45-64) at 25.9%, the young (ages 1-17) at 13.6%, ages 65-84 at 10.3%, and ages 85+ at 1.5%. Chronic ethmoidal sinusitis is more prevalent in the South at 47.6% and the Midwest at 24.9%, followed by the Northeast at 14.0%, and the West at 13.5%.

TABLE 11

Patient and hospital characteristics for ICD-9-CM first-listed diagnosis
code 461.3 Acute Sphenoidal Sinusitis

		All ED visits (those that resulted in admission to the hospital and those that did not)	Only hospital visits that originated in the ED	Only ED visits that ended in discharge (no hospital admission)	Standard errors		
					All ED Visits	Admitted to the hospital from the ED	Discharged from the ED
All discharges		1,410 (100.00%)	238 (100.00%)	1,172 (100.00%)	110	34	101
Age (mean)		45.23	59.92	42.24	1.60	1.60	1.60
Age group	1-17	160 (11.34%)	*	155 (96.92%)	28	*	28 (3.04%)
	18-44	595 (42.19%)	62 (10.50%)	532 (89.50%)	63	16 (2.73%)	62 (2.73%)
	45-64	295 (20.91%)	*	251 (85.04%)	38	*	36 (4.46%)
	65-84	276 (19.54%)	106 (38.38%)	170 (61.62%)	47	24 (7.59%)	39 (7.59%)
	85+	85 (6.01%)	*	*	21	*	*
Sex	Male	434 (30.76%)	77 (17.75%)	357 (82.25%)	52	19 (3.91%)	47 (3.91%)
	Female	976 (69.24%)	161 (16.52%)	815 (83.48%)	86	27 (2.62%)	80 (2.62%)
Median income for zipcode	Low	303 (21.46%)	*	258 (85.40%)	45	*	43 (4.30%)
	Not low	1,048 (74.34%)	175 (16.66%)	874 (83.34%)	91	29 (2.51%)	83 (2.51%)
	Missing	59 (4.20%)	*	*	16	*	*
Region	Northeast	187 (13.27%)	*	136 (72.87%)	32	*	30 (7.90%)
	Midwest	283 (20.05%)	57 (20.20%)	226 (79.80%)	45	16 (5.22%)	41 (5.22%)
	South	630 (44.71%)	102 (16.25%)	528 (83.75%)	79	22 (3.16%)	72 (3.16%)
	West	310 (21.97%)	*	282 (90.99%)	52	*	49 (3.49%)

*Denotes missing values   HCUP-2008

Acute sphenoidal sinusitis is more prevalent in females at 69.2%, and is also seen more in the prime-age group (ages 18-44) at 42.2%, followed by older adults (ages 45-64) at 20.9%, ages 65-84 at 19.5%, and then the young (ages 1-17) at 11.3%, and ages 85+ at 6.0%. Acute sphenoidal sinusitis is more prevalent in the South at 44.7% and the West at 22%, followed by the Midwest at 20.1%, and the Northeast at 13.3%.

TABLE 12

Patient and hospital characteristics for ICD-9-CM first-listed diagnosis code 473.3 Chronic Sphenoidal Sinusitis

		All ED visits (those that resulted in admission to the hospital and those that did not)	Only hospital visits that originated in the ED	Only ED visits that ended in discharge (no hospital admission)	Standard errors		
					All ED Visits	Admitted to the hospital from the ED	Discharged from the ED
All discharges		1,966 (100.00%)	281 (100.00%)	1,685 (100.00%)	125	39	117
Age (mean)		43.75	57.85	41.39	1.15	1.15	1.15
Age group	1-17	224 (11.41%)	*	203 (90.46%)	35	*	32 (4.78%)
	18-44	872 (44.37%)	65 (7.47%)	807 (92.53%)	77	19 (2.03%)	73 (2.03%)
	45-64	439 (22.34%)	*	387 (88.18%)	50	*	47 (3.53%)
	65-84	369 (18.77%)	115 (31.24%)	254 (68.76%)	43	21 (4.87%)	36 (4.87%)
	85+	61 (3.11%)	*	*	17	*	*
Sex	Male	585 (29.75%)	81 (13.84%)	504 (86.16%)	57	22 (3.42%)	52 (3.42%)
	Female	1,381 (70.25%)	201 (14.52%)	1,181 (85.48%)	99	32 (2.18%)	92 (2.18%)
Median income for zipcode	Low	484 (24.62%)	78 (16.11%)	406 (83.89%)	54	22 (4.22%)	50 (4.22%)
	Not low	1,452 (73.84%)	196 (13.48%)	1,256 (86.52%)	109	33 (2.11%)	101 (2.11%)
	Missing	*	*	*	*	*	*
Region	Northeast	226 (11.47%)	*	189 (83.60%)	44	*	41 (6.29%)
	Midwest	487 (24.79%)	56 (11.53%)	431 (88.47%)	60	16 (3.24%)	57 (3.24%)
	South	987 (50.19%)	157 (15.91%)	830 (84.09%)	90	28 (2.67%)	84 (2.67%)
	West	267 (13.55%)	*	235 (88.25%)	46	*	42 (5.26%)

*Denotes missing values   HCUP-2008

Chronic sphenoidal sinusitis is more prevalent in females at 70.3%, and is also seen more in the prime-age group (ages 18-44) at 44.4%, followed by older adults (ages 45-64) at 22.3%, ages 65-84 at 18.8%, the young (ages 1-17) at 11.4%, and ages 85+ at 3.1%. Chronic sphenoidal sinusitis is more prevalent in the South at 50.2% and the Midwest at 24.8%, followed by the West at 13.6%, and the Northeast at 11.5%.

TABLE 13

Patient and hospital characteristics for ICD-9-CM first-listed diagnosis code 461.8 Other Acute Sinusitis

| | | All ED visits (those that resulted in admission to the hospital and those that did not) | Only hospital visits that originated in the ED | Only ED visits that ended in discharge (no hospital admission) | Standard errors | | |
					All ED Visits	Admitted to the hospital from the ED	Discharged from the ED
All discharges		10,999 (100.00%)	974 (100.00%)	10,025 (100.00%)	1,893	104	1,881
Age (mean)		34.92	43.99	34.03	0.79	0.79	0.79
Age group	<1	*			*	*	*
	1-17	1,563 (14.21%)	181 (11.61%)	1,382 (88.39%)	334	38 (3.09%)	328 (3.09%)
	18-44	6,395 (58.14%)	327 (5.11%)	6,068 (94.89%)	1,164	61 (1.29%)	1,162 (1.29%)
	45-64	2,172 (19.75%)	210 (9.66%)	1,962 (90.34%)	374	34 (1.99%)	367 (1.99%)
	65-84	719 (6.54%)	213 (29.64%)	506 (70.36%)	100	34 (5.06%)	93 (5.06%)
	85+	65 (0.59%)	*	*	17	*	*
Sex	Male	4,051 (36.83%)	418 (10.31%)	3,634 (89.69%)	662	55 (1.98%)	655 (1.98%)
	Female	6,948 (63.17%)	557 (8.01%)	6,391 (91.99%)	1,248	69 (1.64%)	1,241 (1.64%)
Median income for zipcode	Low	3,210 (29.18%)	186 (5.80%)	3,023 (94.20%)	818	36 (1.76%)	815 (1.76%)
	Not low	7,432 (67.57%)	715 (9.62%)	6,717 (90.38%)	1,433	75 (1.98%)	1,425 (1.98%)
	Missing	358 (3.25%)	*	284 (79.47%)	81	*	75 (7.04%)
Region	Northeast	*	289 (8.92%)	*	*	72 (3.44%)	*
	Midwest	900 (8.19%)	186 (20.71%)	714 (79.29%)	134	30 (3.70%)	127 (3.70%)
	South	6,113 (55.58%)	365 (5.97%)	5,748 (94.03%)	1,578	58 (1.62%)	1,566 (1.62%)
	West	743 (6.75%)	134 (17.98%)	609 (82.02%)	162	38 (5.83%)	159 (5.83%)

*Denotes missing values   HCUP-2008

Other acute sinusitis is more prevalent in females at 63.2%, and is also seen more in the prime-age group (ages 18-44) at 58.1%, followed by older adults (ages 45-64) at 19.8%, the young (ages 1-17) at 14.2%, ages 65-84 at 6.5%, and ages 85+ at 0.6%. Other acute sinusitis is more prevalent in the South at 55.6% and the Midwest at 8.2%, followed by the West at 6.8%. There was no report for the Northeast in 2008.

TABLE 14

Patient and hospital characteristics for ICD-9-CM first-listed diagnosis code 473.8 Chronic Sinusitis Nec

		All ED visits (those that resulted in admission to the hospital and those that did not)	Only hospital visits that originated in the ED	Only ED visits that ended in discharge (no hospital admission)	Standard errors		
					All ED Visits	Admitted to the hospital from the ED	Discharged from the ED
All discharges		7,886 (100.00%)	757 (100.00%)	7,129 (100.00%)	1,274	112	1,258
Age (mean)		33.30	38.49	32.74	2.05	2.05	2.05
Age group	<1	*		*	*		*
	1-17	*	259 (13.63%)	*	*	76 (5.13%)	*
	18-44	3,573 (45.31%)	168 (4.69%)	3,406 (95.31%)	548	31 (1.03%)	544 (1.03%)
	45-64	1,700 (21.55%)	170 (10.01%)	1,529 (89.99%)	209	40 (2.43%)	204 (2.43%)
	65-84	538 (6.82%)	129 (23.95%)	409 (76.05%)	62	25 (4.58%)	58 (4.58%)
	85+	102 (1.30%)	*	71 (68.96%)	21	*	18 (10.05%)
Sex	Male	3,393 (43.03%)	388 (11.43%)	3,005 (88.57%)	533	76 (2.54%)	521 (2.54%)
	Female	4,493 (56.97%)	369 (8.22%)	4,124 (91.78%)	762	50 (1.66%)	756 (1.66%)
Median income for zipcode	Low	2,935 (37.21%)	192 (6.56%)	2,742 (93.44%)	670	50 (1.96%)	659 (1.96%)
	Not low	4,759 (60.35%)	544 (11.43%)	4,216 (88.57%)	645	76 (2.02%)	637 (2.02%)
	Missing	192 (2.44%)	*	*	53	*	*
Region	Northeast	*	117 (7.70%)	*	*	31 (3.07%)	*
	Midwest	1,409 (17.86%)	106 (7.53%)	1,302 (92.47%)	212	23 (1.79%)	208 (1.79%)
	South	3,907 (49.54%)	410 (10.50%)	*	1,131	98 (3.52%)	*
	West	1,054 (13.36%)	*	930 (88.25%)	282	*	277 (4.27%)

*Denotes missing values   HCUP-2008

Chronic sinusitis Nec is more prevalent in females at 57%, and is also seen more in the prime-age group (ages 18-44) at 45.3%, followed by older adults (ages 45-64) at 21.6%, and ages 65-84 at 6.8%. Chronic sinusitis Nec is more prevalent in the South at 49.5% and the Midwest at 17.9%, followed by the West at 13.4%. There was no report for the Northeast in 2008.

TABLE 15

Patient and hospital characteristics for ICD-9-CM first-listed diagnosis code 461.9 Acute Sinusitis Nos

		All ED visits (those that resulted in admission to the hospital and those that did not)	Only hospital visits that originated in the ED	Only ED visits that ended in discharge (no hospital admission)	Standard errors		
					All ED Visits	Admitted to the hospital from the ED	Discharged from the ED
All discharges		348,238 (100.00%)	2,203 (100.00%)	346,034 (100.00%)	19,179	153	19,165
Age (mean)		34.28	51.71	34.17	0.23	0.23	0.23
Age group	<1	3,421 (0.98%)	*	3,397 (99.30%)	418	*	416 (0.28%)
	1-17	52,527 (15.08%)	256 (0.49%)	52,271 (99.51%)	3,556	37 (0.08%)	3,552 (0.08%)
	18-44	196,773 (56.51%)	499 (0.25%)	196,274 (99.75%)	10,720	67 (0.04%)	10,716 (0.04%)
	45-64	74,691 (21.45%)	630 (0.84%)	74,061 (99.16%)	4,349	63 (0.09%)	4,342 (0.09%)
	65-84	18,867 (5.42%)	637 (3.37%)	18,231 (96.63%)	1,113	61 (0.36%)	1,106 (0.36%)
	85+	1,958 (0.56%)	157 (8.00%)	1,801 (92.00%)	135	26 (1.29%)	131 (1.29%)
Sex	Male	127,162 (36.52%)	968 (0.76%)	126,194 (99.24%)	7,172	88 (0.08%)	7,165 (0.08%)
	Female	221,045 (63.48%)	1,236 (0.56%)	219,809 (99.44%)	12,094	92 (0.05%)	12,087 (0.05%)
	Missing	*		*	*		*
Median income for zipcode	Low	121,933 (35.01%)	670 (0.55%)	121,263 (99.45%)	8,990	85 (0.08%)	8,984 (0.08%)
	Not low	218,496 (62.74%)	1,441 (0.66%)	217,055 (99.34%)	13,078	107 (0.06%)	13,055 (0.06%)
	Missing	7,809 (2.24%)	*	7,716 (98.81%)	582	*	581 (0.37%)
Region	Northeast	52,339 (15.03%)	459 (0.88%)	51,880 (99.12%)	5,257	100 (0.21%)	5,255 (0.21%)
	Midwest	100,758 (28.93%)	516 (0.51%)	100,242 (99.49%)	15,648	59 (0.09%)	15,641 (0.09%)
	South	162,959 (46.80%)	989 (0.61%)	161,970 (99.39%)	9,415	88 (0.06%)	9,400 (0.06%)
	West	32,182 (9.24%)	240 (0.75%)	31,942 (99.25%)	2,586	44 (0.14%)	2,582 (0.14%)

*Denotes missing values   HCUP-2008

Acute sinusitis Nos is more prevalent in females at 63.5%, and is also seen more in the prime-age group (ages 18-44) at 56.5%, followed by older adults (ages 45-64) at 21.5%, then the young (ages 1-17) at 15.1%, and finally, ages 65-84 at 5.42%. Acute sinusitis Nos is more prevalent in the South at 46.8% and the Midwest at 28.9%, followed by the Northeast at 15.0%, and the West at 9.2%.

TABLE 16

Patient and hospital characteristics for ICD-9-CM first-listed diagnosis code 473.9 Chronic Sinusitis Nos

		All ED visits (those that resulted in admission to the hospital and those that did not)	Only hospital visits that originated in the ED	Only ED visits that ended in discharge (no hospital admission)	Standard errors		
					All ED Visits	Admitted to the hospital from the ED	Discharged from the ED
All discharges		332,400 (100.00%)	2,219 (100.00%)	330,181 (100.00%)	23,712	190	23,675
Age (mean)		33.58	45.03	33.51	0.26	0.26	0.26
Age group	<1	3,736 (1.12%)	*	3,689 (98.73%)	298	*	297 (0.46%)
	1-17	60,812 (18.29%)	494 (0.81%)	60,319 (99.19%)	5,273	109 (0.18%)	5,252 (0.18%)
	18-44	176,437 (53.08%)	423 (0.24%)	176,014 (99.76%)	12,548	55 (0.03%)	12,538 (0.03%)
	45-64	70,869 (21.32%)	643 (0.91%)	70,226 (99.09%)	5,120	72 (0.11%)	5,109 (0.11%)
	65-84	18,401 (5.54%)	466 (2.53%)	17,935 (97.47%)	1,163	46 (0.28%)	1,158 (0.28%)
	85+	2,134 (0.64%)	145 (6.78%)	1,989 (93.22%)	151	27 (1.26%)	148 (1.26%)
	Missing	*		*	*		*
Sex	Male	124,544 (37.47%)	973 (0.78%)	123,571 (99.22%)	8,549	104 (0.09%)	8,529 (0.09%)
	Female	207,830 (62.52%)	1,245 (0.60%)	206,584 (99.40%)	15,230	119 (0.07%)	15,211 (0.07%)
	Missing	*		*	*		*
Median income for zipcode	Low	121,643 (36.60%)	640 (0.53%)	121,004 (99.47%)	11,570	91 (0.08%)	11,556 (0.08%)
	Not low	202,786 (61.01%)	1,494 (0.74%)	201,292 (99.26%)	13,418	138 (0.07%)	13,386 (0.07%)
	Missing	7,970 (2.40%)	85 (1.07%)	7,885 (98.93%)	675	23 (0.28%)	671 (0.28%)
Region	Northeast	44,269 (13.32%)	520 (1.17%)	43,750 (98.83%)	4,399	95 (0.23%)	4,387 (0.23%)
	Midwest	110,316 (33.19%)	481 (0.44%)	109,834 (99.56%)	21,732	78 (0.10%)	21,712 (0.10%)
	South	141,566 (42.59%)	999 (0.71%)	140,567 (99.29%)	7,912	139 (0.09%)	7,861 (0.09%)
	West	36,249 (10.91%)	219 (0.60%)	36,030 (99.40%)	2,841	42 (0.12%)	2,834 (0.12%)

*Denotes missing values   HCUP-2008

Chronic sinusitis Nos is more prevalent in females at 62.5%, and is also seen more in the prime-age group (ages 18-44) at 53.1%, followed by older adults (ages 45-64) at 21.3%, the young (ages 1-17) at 18.3%, and ages 65-84 at 5.5%. Chronic sinusitis is more prevalent in the South at 42.6% and the Midwest at 33.2%, followed by the Northeast at 13.3%, and the West at 10.9%.

TABLE 17

Patient and hospital characteristics for ICD-9-CM first-listed diagnosis code 372.00 Acute Conjunctivitis Nos

		All ED visits (those that resulted in admission to the hospital and those that did not)	Only hospital visits that originated in the ED	Only ED visits that ended in discharge (no hospital admission)	Standard errors		
					All ED Visits	Admitted to the hospital from the ED	Discharged from the ED
All discharges		101,249 (100.00%)	114 (100.00%)	101,134 (100.00%)	6,327	26	6,330
Age (mean)		20.90	26.70	20.89	0.64	0.64	0.64
Age group	<1	9,843 (9.72%)	*	9,800 (99.57%)	837	*	841 (0.20%)
	1-17	41,166 (40.66%)	*	41,144 (99.95%)	3,432	*	3,432 (0.02%)
	18-44	35,365 (34.93%)	*	35,354 (99.97%)	2,168	*	2,168 (0.02%)
	45-64	11,515 (11.37%)	*	11,487 (99.76%)	727	*	726 (0.10%)
	65-84	2,958 (2.92%)	*	2,954 (99.89%)	206	*	206 (0.11%)
	85+	402 (0.40%)	*	395 (98.22%)	47	*	47 (1.27%)
Sex	Male	46,980 (46.40%)	48 (0.10%)	46,932 (99.90%)	3,081	14 (0.03%)	3,083 (0.03%)
	Female	54,257 (53.59%)	66 (0.12%)	54,190 (99.88%)	3,306	19 (0.04%)	3,307 (0.04%)
	Missing	*		*	*	*	*
Median income for zipcode	Low	30,493 (30.12%)	*	30,459 (99.89%)	3,100	*	3,101 (0.04%)
	Not low	68,891 (68.04%)	*	68,821 (99.90%)	4,710	*	4,713 (0.03%)
	Missing	1,865 (1.84%)	*	1,855 (99.46%)	172	*	172 (0.38%)
Region	Northeast	30,960 (30.58%)	*	30,921 (99.87%)	4,074	*	4,078 (0.07%)
	Midwest	23,220 (22.93%)	*	23,202 (99.92%)	3,344	*	3,345 (0.04%)
	South	30,396 (30.02%)	*	30,353 (99.86%)	2,924	*	2,925 (0.05%)
	West	16,673 (16.47%)	*	16,658 (99.91%)	1,923	*	1,921 (0.05%)

*Denotes missing values　　　　　　　　　　　　　　HCUP-2008

Acute conjunctivitis Nos is more prevalent in females at 54%, and is also seen more in the young (ages 1-17) at 40.7%, followed by the prime-age group (ages 18-44) at 34.9%, the older adults (ages 45-64) at 11.4%, ages 65-84 at 2.9%, those younger than one year old at 9.7%, and finally, the 85+ age group at 0.4%. Acute conjunctivitis Nos is more prevalent in the Northeast at 30.6%, followed by the South at 30.0%, the Midwest at 22.9%, and the West at 16.5%.

TABLE 18

Patient and hospital characteristics for ICD-9-CM first-listed diagnosis code 372.30 Chronic Conjunctivitis Nos

		All ED visits (those that resulted in admission to the hospital and those that did not)	Only hospital visits that originated in the ED	Only ED visits that ended in discharge (no hospital admission)	All ED Visits	Standard errors		
						Admitted to the hospital from the ED	Discharged from the ED	
All discharges		377,933 (100.00%)	282 (100.00%)	377,651 (100.00%)	12,513	66	12,505	
Age (mean)		21.68	31.01	21.67	0.35	0.35	0.35	
Age group	<1	35,899 (9.50%)	*	35,834 (99.82%)	1,807	*	1,804 (0.06%)	
	1-17	145,562 (38.52%)	56 (0.04%)	145,506 (99.96%)	6,349	16 (0.01%)	6,347 (0.01%)	
	18-44	138,489 (36.64%)	*	138,425 (99.95%)	4,662	*	4,662 (0.03%)	
	45-64	44,668 (11.82%)	*	44,626 (99.91%)	1,485	*	1,485 (0.03%)	
	65-84	11,453 (3.03%)	*	11,411 (99.63%)	435	*	432 (0.11%)	
	85+	1,858 (0.49%)	*	1,845 (99.29%)	105	*	104 (0.41%)	
	Missing	*		*	*		*	
Sex	Male	174,112 (46.07%)	*	174,006 (99.94%)	5,832	*	5,829 (0.02%)	
	Female	203,792 (53.92%)	176 (0.09%)	203,616 (99.91%)	6,799	41 (0.02%)	6,795 (0.02%)	
	Missing	*		*	*		*	
Median income for zipcode	Low	134,542 (35.60%)	*	134,396 (99.89%)	6,847	*	6,844 (0.04%)	
	Not low	234,789 (62.12%)	132 (0.06%)	234,657 (99.94%)	8,705	26 (0.01%)	8,699 (0.01%)	
	Missing	8,601 (2.28%)	*	8,598 (99.96%)	691	*	690 (0.04%)	
Region	Northeast	69,312 (18.34%)	*	69,220 (99.87%)	5,634	*	5,630 (0.04%)	
	Midwest	104,777 (27.72%)	*	104,752 (99.98%)	6,819	*	6,819 (0.01%)	
	South	144,513 (38.24%)	*	144,371 (99.90%)	7,794	*	7,785 (0.04%)	
	West	59,330 (15.70%)	*	59,308 (99.96%)	4,193	*	4,190 (0.02%)	

*Denotes missing values   HCUP-2008

Chronic conjunctivitis Nos is more prevalent in females at 54%, and is also seen more in the young (ages 1-17) at 38.5%, followed by the prime-age group (ages 18-44) at 36.6%, the older adults (ages 45-64) at 11.8%, those younger than one year old at 9.5%, ages 65-84 at 3.0%, and ages 85+ at 0.5%. Chronic conjunctivitis Nos is more prevalent in the South at 38.2%, followed by the Midwest at 27.7%, then the Northeast at 18.3%, and the West at 15.7%.

TABLE 19

Patient and hospital characteristics for ICD-9-CM first-listed diagnosis code 372.14 Chronic Allergic Conjunctivitis Nec

		All ED visits (those that resulted in admission to the hospital and those that did not)	Only hospital visits that originated in the ED	Only ED visits that ended in discharge (no hospital admission)	All ED Visits	Admitted to the hospital from the ED	Discharged from the ED
						Standard errors	
All discharges		36,456 (100.00%)	*	36,433 (100.00%)	1,527	*	1,526
Age (mean)		24.78	*	24.77	0.55	*	0.55
Age group	<1	439 (1.20%)		439 (100.00%)	51		51 (0.00%)
	1-17	15,851 (43.48%)	*	15,841 (99.94%)	1,039	*	1,039 (0.05%)
	18-44	13,617 (37.35%)		13,617 (100.00%)	586		586 (0.00%)
	45-64	5,169 (14.18%)	*	5,166 (99.94%)	262	*	262 (0.06%)
	65-84	1,252 (3.44%)	*	1,247 (99.57%)	91	*	91 (0.43%)
	85+	128 (0.35%)	*	124 (96.68%)	25	*	25 (3.29%)
Sex	Male	17,526 (48.08%)		17,526 (100.00%)	814		814 (0.00%)
	Female	18,925 (51.91%)	*	18,902 (99.88%)	800	*	799 (0.05%)
	Missing	*		*	*		*
Median income for zipcode	Low	12,980 (35.61%)	*	12,973 (99.94%)	932	*	932 (0.04%)
	Not low	22,876 (62.75%)	*	22,866 (99.96%)	1,037	*	1,037 (0.03%)
	Missing	599 (1.64%)	*	594 (99.10%)	71	*	72 (0.91%)
Region	Northeast	9,181 (25.19%)	*	9,166 (99.84%)	895	*	894 (0.09%)
	Midwest	8,745 (23.99%)	*	8,741 (99.95%)	661	*	660 (0.05%)
	South	13,287 (36.45%)	*	13,284 (99.98%)	952	*	952 (0.02%)
	West	5,242 (14.38%)		5,242 (100.00%)	431		431 (0.00%)

*Denotes missing values   HCUP-2008

Chronic allergic conjunctivitis Nec is more prevalent in females at 52%, and is also seen more in the young (ages 1-17) at 43.5%, followed by the prime-age group (ages 18-44) at 37.4%, the older adults (ages 45-64) at 14.2%, ages 65-84 at 3.4%, those younger than one year old at 1.2%, and ages 85+ at 0.4%. Chronic allergic conjunctivitis Nec is more prevalent in the South at 36.5%, followed by the Northeast at 25.2%, then the Midwest at 24%, and the West at 14.4%.

BIBLIOGRAPHICAL NOTES

Chapter 1: ALLERGIC RHINITIS, SINUSITIS, AND CONJUNCTIVITIS ED DISCHARGES

The HCUP statistics are obtained from data published at: http://hcupnet.ahrq.gov/

HCUPnet is a free, online query system based on data from the Healthcare Cost and Utilization Project (HCUP). It provides access to health statistics and information on hospital inpatient and emergency department utilization.

http://water.usgs.gov/nawqa/pnsp/usage/maps/

Epstein, Samuel S., Randall Fitzgerald. 2009. *Toxic Beauty: How Cosmetics and Personal Care Products Endanger Your Health... And What You Can Do About It.* Ben Bella Books

Ruth Winter. 2009. *A Consumer's Dictionary of Cosmetic Ingredients, 7th Edition: Complete Information About the Harmful and Desirable Ingredients Found in Cosmetics and Cosmeceuticals.* New York: Three Rivers Press

Chapter 2: ALLERGY IN CHILDHOOD

aaaai.org, acaai.org

Chapter 3: ESTROGEN EPIDEMIC AND ADULT-ONSET RHINITIS

Definition of RBL-2H3 found at the beginning of Chapter 3:

(RBL-2H3 is a basophilic leukemia cell line isolated and cloned in 1978, in the Laboratory of Immunology at the National Institute of Dental Research, from Wistar rat basophilic cells that were maintained as tumors. These cells have high affinity IgE receptors. They can be activated to secrete histamine and other mediators by aggregation of these receptors or with calcium ionophores. They have been used extensively to study FcERI and the biochemical pathways for secretion in mast cells. See www.atcc.org).

Prevention of severe premenstrual asthma attacks by leukotriene receptor antagonist

Hiroko Nakasato MD, Takashi Ohrui MD, Kiyohisa Sekizawa MD, Toshifumi Matsui MD, Mutsuo Yamaya MD, Gen Tamura MD, Hidetada Sasaki MD

The Department of Geriatric Medicine Sendai, Japan The First Department of Internal Medicine, Tohoku University School of Medicine, Sendai, Japan

Abstract

Background: The etiology and treatment of premenstrual exacerbations of asthma (PMA) remain uncertain. **Objective:** We investigated the role of cellular mediators released from inflammatory cells in the airflow limitation during PMA. **Methods:** Serum levels of leukotriene (LT) B_4 , LTC_4 , platelet-activating factor, histamine, IL-1β, IL-4, IL-5, IL-6, and GM-CSF were measured at different time points, first just before or during menstruation when the peak expiratory flow rate (PEFR) began to decrease precipitously and second during the menstrual midcycle week (days 10-16) when the PEFR returned to baseline values in patients with PMA and in age-matched asthma patients without PMA at the same intervals. **Results:** Serum levels of LTC_4 were significantly higher during exacerbations of asthma than after recovery (69.0 ± 16.0 pg/mL vs. 24.0 ± 9.5 pg/mL, $P < .05$), whereas those of IL-1β, IL-4, IL-5, IL-6, GM-CSF, histamine, LTB_4, and platelet-activating factor did not differ between 2 periods in 5 patients with PMA. In contrast, in 5 asthmatic patients without PMA serum levels of cellular mediators did not differ between corresponding periods. Oral administration of pranlukast, an LT receptor antagonist (225 mg twice daily), significantly reduced decreases in PEFR from the baseline values (110 ± 21 L/min with pranlukast vs. 233 ± 20 L/min without pranlukast, $P < .01$) in association with an improvement of asthma symptom scores (6.5 ± 1.1 with pranlukast vs. 9.8 ± 0.7 without pranlukast, $P < 0.05$) in 5 patients with PMA. **Conclusion:** LTs are partly involved in the pathogenesis of PMA, and LT receptor antagonists may be useful for preventing airflow obstruction in patients with PMA. (J Allergy Clin Immunol 1999; 104:585-8.)

The estrogen effect on mast cells is captured in the following articles and their references.

Variables in Allergy Skin Testing

Immunology and Allergy Clinics of North America — *Volume 21, Issue 2* (May 2001)

Harold S. Nelson MD

Department of Medicine, National Jewish Medical and Research Center, Denver, Colorado

Address reprint requests to
Harold S. Nelson, MD
National Jewish Medical and Research Center
1400 Jackson Street
Denver, CO 80206
e-mail: nelsonh@njc.org

Skin testing is usually the preferred method for the diagnosis of immunoglobulin E (IgE)-mediated hypersensitivity because it is simple, inexpensive, and the results are immediately available. Like any laboratory test, however, a number of variables can affect the outcome, such as:

Variations with the Menstrual Cycle

Skin test reactions to histamine and allergen vary in women with their menstrual cycle. [1] Reactions to both are larger in midcycle (days 12-16) than during the menses (day 1-4) or the late progesterone phase (days 24-28).

Reference:

1. Kalogeromitros D, Katsarou A, Armenaka M, et al.: Influence of the menstrual cycle on skin-prick test reactions to histamine, morphine and allergens. Clin Exp Allergy 25:461-465, 1995

Influence of the menstrual cycle on skin-prick test reactions to histamine, morphine and allergen. Kalogeromitros D. *Clin Exp Allergy* 1 May 1995; 25(5): 461-6

Abstract:

The purpose of this study was to examine the possible influence of the phases of the menstrual cycle on dermal reactivity to skin-prick testing. We studied 15 atopic, menstruating women with seasonal rhinoconjunctivitis and/or asthma, with known sensitivity to olive and Parietaria (mean age 25.2 years) and 15 non-atopic, healthy, female controls (mean age 24.7 years). Skin-prick tests with histamine, morphine, and in the atopic group with Parietaria/and/or olive, were repeated three times during the same menstrual cycle, corresponding to bleeding (day 1-4), midcycle (day 12-16), and the late progesterone phase (day 24-28). None of the patients had received oral antihistamines or exogenous hormones for at least 1 month prior to testing. Results indicate a significant increase in weal-and-flare size to histamine, morphine, and Parietaria on days 12-16 of the cycle, corresponding to ovulation and peak estrogen levels. This was observed in both atopic and non-atopic women. Differences in skin reactivity to histamine and morphine between the groups were not significant. Therefore, in women, the phase of the menstrual cycle is another factor that may influence skin-test results.

Estradiol activates mast cells via a non-genomic estrogen receptor-α and calcium influx.

Zaitsu M, Narita S, Lambert KC, Grady JJ, Estes DM, et al. 2007. "Estradiol activates mast cells via a non-genomic estrogen receptor-alpha and calcium influx." Mol Immunol 44(8): 1977-85.

References:

Barr RG, Wentowski CC, Grodstein F, Somers SC, Stampfer MJ, Schwartz J, Speizer FE, Camargo CA, Jr. Prospective study of postmenopausal hormone use and newly diagnosed asthma and chronic obstructive pulmonary disease. Arch Intern Med 2004; 164:379-386. [Pub Med: 14980988]

Bulayeva NN, Gametchu B, Watson CS. Quantitative measurement of estrogen-induced ERK 1 and 2 activation via multiple membrane-initiated signaling pathways. Steroids 2004; 69:181-192. [Pub Med: 15072920]

Bulayeva NN, Wozniak AL, Lash LL, Watson CS. Mechanisms of membrane estrogen receptor-alpha mediated rapid stimulation of Ca2+ levels and prolactin release in a pituitary cell line. Am J Physiology Endocrinol Metab 2005; 288:E388-E397. [Pub Med: 15494610]

Butterfield JH, Weiler D, Dewald G, Gleich GJ. Establishment of an immature mast cell line from a patient with mast cell leukemia. Leuk Res 1988; 12:345-355. [Pub Med: 3131594]

Cary, NC. SAS Publishing. 2000.

Cocchiara R, Albeggiani G, Di Trapani G, Azzolina A, Lampiasi N, Rizzo F, Diotallevi L, Gianaroli L, Geraci D. Oestradiol enhances in vitro the histamine release induced by embryonic histamine-releasing factor (EHRF) from uterine mast cells. Hum Reprod 1992; 7:1036-1041. [Pub Med: 1383260]

Cocchiara R, Albeggiani G, Di Trapani G, Azzolina A, Lampiasi N, Rizzo F, Geraci D. Modulation of rat peritoneal mast cell and human basophil histamine release by estrogens. Int Arch Allergy Appl Immunol 1990; 93:192-197. [Pub Med: 1712002]

Collins P, Webb C. Estrogen hits the surface. Nat Med 1999; 5:1130-1131. [Pub Med: 10502813]

Dastych J, Walczak-Drzewiecka A, Wyczolkowska J, Metcalfe DD. Murine mast cells exposed to mercuric chloride release granule-associated N-acetyl-beta-D-hexosaminidase and secrete IL-4 and TNF-alpha. J Allergy Clin Immunol 1999; 103:1108-1114. [Pub Med: 10359893]

De Marco R, Locatelli F, Cerveri I, Bugiani M, Marinoni A, Giammanco G. Incidence and remission of asthma: a retrospective study on the natural history of asthma in Italy. J Allergy Clin Immunol 2002; 110:228-235. [Pub Med: 12170262]

Dijkstra A, Howard TD, Vonk JM, Ampleford EJ, Lange LA, Bleecker ER, Meyers DA, Postma DS. Estrogen receptor 1 polymorphisms are associated with airway hyperresponsiveness and lung function decline, particularly in female subjects with asthma. J Allergy Clin Immunol 2006; 117:604-611. [Pub Med: 16522460]

Doolan CM, Condliffe SB, Harvey BJ. Rapid non-genomic activation of cytosolic cyclic AMP-dependent protein kinase activity and [Ca(2+)](i) by 17-beta-oestradiol in female rat distal colon. Br J Pharmacol 2000; 129:1375-1386. [Pub Med: 10742293]

Doolan CM, Harvey BJ. A Galphas protein-coupled membrane receptor, distinct from the classical estrogen receptor, transduces rapid effects of oestradiol on [Ca2+]i in female rat distal colon. Mol Cell Endocrinol 2003; 199:87-103. [Pub Med: 12581882]

Durstin M, Durstin S, Molski TF, Becker EL, Sha'afi RI. Cytoplasmic phospholipase A2 translocates to membrane fraction in human neutrophils activated by stimuli that phosphorylate mitogen-activated protein kinase. Proc Natl Acad Sci USA 1994; 91:3142-3146. [Pub Med: 7512725]

Fiorini S, Ferretti ME, Biondi C, Pavan B, Lunghi L, Paganetto G, Abelli L. 17Beta-estradiol stimulates arachidonate release from human amnion-like WISH cells through a rapid mechanism involving a membrane receptor. Endocrinology 2003; 144:3359-3367. [Pub Med: 12865314]

Harnish DC, Albert LM, Leathurby Y, Eckert AM, Ciarletta A, Kasaian M, Keith JC, Jr. Beneficial effects of estrogen treatment in the HLA-B27 transgenic rat model of inflammatory bowel disease. Am J Physiology Gastrointest Liver Physiology 2004; 286:G118-G125. [Pub Med: 12958017]

Improta-Brears T, Whorton AR, Codazzi F, York JD, Meyer T, McDonnell DP. Estrogen-induced activation of mitogen-activated protein kinase requires mobilization of intracellular calcium. Proc Natl Acad Sci USA 1999; 96:4686-4691. [Pub Med: 10200323]

Ishizaka T, Hirata F, Ishizaka K, Axelrod J. Stimulation of phospholipid methylation, Ca2+ influx, and histamine release by bridging of IgE receptors on rat mast cells. Proc Natl Acad Sci USA 1980; 77:1903-1906. [Pub Med: 6154940]

Jiang YA, Zhang YY, Luo HS, Xing SF. Mast cell density and the context of clinicopathological parameters and expression of p185, estrogen receptor, and proliferating cell nuclear antigen in gastric carcinoma. World J Gastroenterol 2002; 8:1005-1008. [Pub Med: 12439914]

Lambert KC, Curran EM, Judy BM, Lubahn DB, Estes DM.

Estrogen receptor-{alpha} deficiency promotes increased TNF-{alpha} secretion and bacterial killing by murine macrophages in response to microbial stimuli in vitro. J Leukoc Biol 2004; 75:1166-1172. [Pub Med: 15020652]

Lambert KC, Curran EM, Judy BM, Milligan GN, Lubahn DB, Estes DM. Estrogen receptor {alpha} (ER{alpha}) deficiency in macrophages results in increased stimulation of CD4+ T cells while 17 {beta}-estradiol acts through ER{alpha} to increase IL-4 and GATA-3 expression in CD4+ T cells independent of antigen presentation. J Immunol 2005; 175:5716-5723. [Pub Med: 16237062]

Mannino DM, Homa DM, Akinbami LJ, Moorman JE, Gwynn C, Redd SC. Surveillance for asthma—United States, 1980-1999. MMWR Surveill Summ 2002; 51:1-13.

Morita Y, Siraganian RP. Inhibition of IgE-mediated histamine release from rat basophilic leukemia cells and rat mast cells by inhibitors of trans-methylation. J Immunol 1981; 127:1339-1344. [Pub Med: 6168684]

Nadal A, Ropero AB, Laribi O, Maillet M, Fuentes E, Soria B. Nongenomic actions of estrogens and xenoestrogens by binding at a plasma membrane receptor unrelated to estrogen receptor alpha and estrogen receptor beta. Proc Natl Acad Sci USA 2000; 97:11603-11608. [Pub Med: 11027358]

Nakasato H, Ohrui T, Sekizawa K, Matsui T, Yamaya M, Tamura G, Sasaki H. Prevention of severe premenstrual asthma attacks by leukotriene receptor antagonist. J Allergy Clin Immunol 1999; 104:585-588. [Pub Med: 10482831]

Nicovani S, Rudolph MI. Estrogen receptors in mast cells from arterial walls. Biocell 2002; 26:15-24. [Pub Med: 12058378]

Odom S, Gomez G, Kovarova M, Furumoto Y, Ryan JJ, Wright HV, Gonzalez-Espinosa C, Hibbs ML, Harder KW, Rivera J. Negative regulation of immunoglobulin E-dependent allergic responses by Lyn kinase. J Exp Med 2004; 199:1491-1502. [Pub Med: 15173205]

Pouliot M, McDonald PP, Krump E, Mancini JA, McColl SR, Weech PK, Borgeat P. Colocalization of cytosolic phospholipase A2, 5-lipoxygenase, and 5-lipoxygenase-activating protein at the nuclear membrane of A23187-stimulated human neutrophils. Eur J Biochem 1996; 238:250-258. [Pub Med: 8665944]

Schatz M, Camargo CA, Jr. The relationship of sex to asthma prevalence, health care utilization, and medications in a large managed-care organization. Ann Allergy Asthma Immunol 2003; 91:553-558. [Pub Med: 14700439]

Simoncini T, Mannella P, Fornari L, Caruso A, Varone G, Genazzani AR. Genomic and non-genomic effects of estrogens on endothelial cells. Steroids 2004; 69:537-542. [Pub Med: 15288766]

Skobeloff EM, Spivey WH, Silverman R, Eskin BA, Harchelroad F, Alessi TV. The effect of the menstrual cycle on asthma presentations in the emergency department. Arch Intern Med 1996; 156:1837-1840. [Pub Med: 8790078]

Skobeloff EM, Spivey WH, St Clair SS, Schoffstall JM. The influence of age and sex on asthma admissions. JAMA 1992; 268:3437-3440. [Pub Med: 1460733]

Smith GD, Lee RJ, Oliver JM, Keizer J. Effect of Ca2+ influx on intracellular free Ca2+ responses in antigen-stimulated RBL-2H3 cells. Am J Physiology 1996; 270:C939-C952. [Pub Med: 8638649]

Song RX, Barnes CJ, Zhang Z, Bao Y, Kumar R, Santen RJ. The role of Shc and insulin-like growth factor 1 receptor in mediating the translocation of estrogen receptor alpha to the plasma membrane. Proc Natl Acad Sci USA 2004; 101:2076-2081. [Pub Med: 14764897]

Spanos C, el-Mansoury M, Letourneau R, Minogiannis P, Greenwood J, Siri P, Sant GR, Theoharides TC. Carbachol-induced bladder mast cell activation: augmentation by estradiol and implications for interstitial cystitis. Urology 1996; 48:809-816. [Pub Med: 8911535]

Stefano GB, Prevot V, Beauvillain JC, Fimiani C, Welters I, Cadet P, Breton C, Pestel J, Salzet M, Bilfinger TV. Estradiol coupling to human monocyte nitric oxide release is dependent on intracellular calcium transients: evidence for an estrogen surface receptor. J Immunol 1999; 163:3758-3763. [Pub Med: 10490972]

Suzuki Y, Yoshimaru T, Matsui T, Inoue T, Niide O, Nunomura S, Ra C. Fc epsilon RI signaling of mast cells activates intracellular production of hydrogen peroxide: role in the regulation of calcium signals. J Immunol 2003; 171:6119-6127. [Pub Med: 14634127]

Vliagoftis H, Dimitriadou V, Boucher W, Rozniecki JJ, Correia I, Raam S, Theoharides TC. Estradiol augments while Tamoxifen inhibits rat mast cell secretion. Int Arch Allergy Immunol 1992;

98:398-409. [Pub Med: 1384869]

Vrieze A, Postma DS, Kerstjens HA. Perimenstrual asthma: a syndrome without known cause or cure. J Allergy Clin Immunol 2003; 112:271-282. [Pub Med: 12897732]

Wang HQ, Kim MP, Tiano HF, Langenbach R, Smart RC. Protein kinase C-alpha coordinately regulates cytosolic phospholipase A (2) activity and the expression of cyclooxygenase-2 through different mechanisms in mouse keratinocytes. Mol Pharmacol 2001; 59:860-866. [Pub Med: 11259631]

Watson CS, Norfleet AM, Pappas TC, Gametchu B. Rapid actions of estrogens in GH3/B6 pituitary tumor cells via a plasma membrane version of estrogen receptor-alpha. Steroids 1999; 64:5-13. [Pub Med: 10323667]

Wozniak AL, Bulayeva NN, Watson CS. Xenoestrogens at picomolar to nanomolar concentrations trigger membrane estrogen receptor-alpha-mediated Ca2+ fluxes and prolactin release in GH3/B6 pituitary tumor cells. Environ Health Perspect 2005; 113:431-439. [Pub Med: 15811834]

Zhao XJ, McKerr G, Dong Z, Higgins CA, Carson J, Yang ZQ, Hannigan BM. Expression of oestrogen and progesterone receptors by mast cells alone, but not lymphocytes, macrophages or other immune cells in human upper airways. Thorax 2001; 56:205-211. [Pub Med: 11182013]

Zivadinovic D, Gametchu B, Watson CS. Membrane estrogen receptor-alpha levels in MCF-7 breast cancer cells predict cAMP and proliferation responses. Breast Cancer Res 2005; 7:R101-R112. [Pub Med: 15642158]

Environmental Estrogens Induce Mast Cell Degranulation and Enhance IgE-Mediated Release of Allergic Mediators

Shin-ichiro Narita[1], Randall M. Goldblum[1], Cheryl S. Watson[2], Edward G. Brooks[1], D. Mark Estes[1], Edward M. Curran[1], and Terumi Midoro-Horiuti[1]

[1]Department of Pediatrics, Child Health Research Center; and [2]Department of Biochemistry and Molecular Biology, University of Texas Medical Branch, Galveston, Texas, USA

References:

Aravindakshan J, Gregory M, Marcogliese DJ, Fournier M, Cyr DG. 2004. Consumption of xenoestrogen-contaminated fish during lactation alters adult male reproductive function. Toxicol Sci 81:179-189.

Ayotte P, Muckle G, Jacobson JL, Jacobson SW, Dewailly É. 2003. Assessment of pre- and postnatal exposure to polychlorinated biphenyls: lessons from the Inuit Cohort Study. Environ Health Perspect 111:1253-1258.

Bologa CG, Revankar CM, Young SM, Edwards BS, Arterburn JB, Kiselyov AS, et al. 2006. Virtual and biomolecular screening converge on a selective agonist for GPR30. Nat Chem Biol 2:207-212.

Bulayeva NN, Watson CS. 2004. Xenoestrogen-induced ERK-1 and ERK-2 activation via multiple membrane-initiated signaling pathways. Environ Health Perspect 112:1481-1487.

Bulayeva NN, Wozniak AL, Lash LL, Watson CS. 2005. Mechanisms of membrane estrogen-α-mediated rapid stimulation of Ca2+ levels and prolactin release in a pituitary cell line. Am J Physiology Endocrinol Metab 288:E388-E397.

Burr ML, Wat D, Evans C, Dunstan FD, Doull IJ. 2006. Asthma prevalence in 1973, 1988, and 2003. Thorax 61:296-299.

Butterfield JH, Weiler D, Dewald G, Gleich GJ. 1988. Establishment of an immature mast cell line from a patient with mast cell leukemia. Leuk Res 12:345-355.

Dastych J, Walczak-Drzewiecka A, Wyczolkowska J, Metcalfe DD. 1999. Murine mast cells exposed to mercuric chloride release granule-associated N-acetyl-β-Dhexosaminidase and secrete IL-4 and TNF-α. J Allergy Clin Immunol 103:1108-1114.

De Marco R, Locatelli F, Cerveri I, Bugiani M, Marinoni A, Giammanco G. 2002. Incidence and remission of asthma: a retrospective study on the natural history of asthma in Italy. J Allergy clin Immunol 110:228-2

Dewailly É, Ayotte P, Bruneau S, Laliberté C, Muir DCG, Norstrom RJ. 1993. Inuit exposure to organochlorines through the aquatic food chain in arctic Quebec. Environ

Health Perspect 101:618-620.

Dijkstra A, Howard TD, Vonk JM, Ampleford EJ, Lange LA, Bleecker ER, et al. 2006. Estrogen receptor 1 polymorphisms are associated with airway hyperresponsiveness and lung function decline, particularly in female subjects with asthma. J Allergy Clin Immunol 117:604-611.

Falconer IR, Chapman HF, Moore MR, Ranmuthugala G. 2006. Endocrine-disrupting compounds: a review of their challenge to sustainable and safe water supply and water

reuse. Environ Toxicol 21:181-191.

Ibarluzea JJ, Fernandez MF, Santa-Marina L, Olea-Serrano MF, Rivas AM, Aurrekoetxea JJ, et al. 2004. Breast cancer risk and the combined effect of environmental estrogens. Cancer Causes Control 15:591-600.

Kos M, Denger S, Reid G, Korach KS, Gannon F. 2002. Down but not out? A novel protein isoform of the estrogen receptor α is expressed in the estrogen receptor α knockout mouse. J Mol Endocrinol 29:281-286.

Lambert KC, Curran EM, Judy BM, Milligan GN, Lubahn DB, Estes DM. 2005. Estrogen receptor α (ERα) deficiency in macrophages results in increased stimulation of CD4+ T cells while 17β-estradiol acts through ERα to increase IL-4 and GATA-3 expression in CD4+ T cells independent of antigen presentation. J Immunol 175:5716-5723.

Metcalfe CD, Metcalfe TL, Kiparissis Y, Koenig BG, Khan C, Hughes RJ, et al. 2001. Estrogenic potency of chemicals detected in sewage treatment plant effluents as determined by in vivo assays with Japanese medaka (Oryzias latipes). Environ Toxicol Chem 20:297-308.

Newbold RR, Padilla-Banks E, Jefferson WN. 2006. Adverse effects of the model environmental estrogen diethylstilbestrol are transmitted to subsequent generations.

Endocrinology 147(suppl 6):S11-S17.

Odom S, Gomez G, Kovarova M, Furumoto Y, Ryan JJ, Wright HV, et al. 2004. Negative regulation of immunoglobulin E-dependent allergic responses by Lyn kinase. J Exp Med 199:1491-1502.

Solomon GM, Weiss PM. 2002. Chemical contaminants in breast milk: time trends and regional variability. Environ Health Perspect 110:A339-A347.

Thomas P, Pang Y, Filardo EJ, Dong J. 2005. Identity of an estrogen membrane receptor coupled to a G protein in human breast cancer cells. Endocrinology 146:624-632.

Vartiainen T, Saarikoski S, Jaakkola JJ, Tuomisto J. 1997. PCDD, PCDF, and PCB concentrations in human milk from two areas in Finland. Chemosphere 34:2571-2583.

Wang SL, Lin CY, Guo YL, Lin LY, Chou WL, Chang LW. 2004. Infant exposure to polychlorinated dibenzo-p-dioxins, dibenzofurans and biphenyls (PCDD/Fs, PCBs)—correlation between prenatal and postnatal exposure. Chemosphere 54:1459-1473.

Watson CS, Campbell CH, Gametchu B. 1999. Membrane oestrogen receptors on rat pituitary tumour cells: immunoidentification and responses to oestradiol and xenoestrogens. Exp Physiology 84:1013-1022.

Watson CS, Gametchu B. 2001. Membrane estrogen and glucocorticoid receptors—implications for hormonal control of immune function and autoimmunity. Int Immunopharmacol 1:1049-1063.

Watson CS, Gametchu B. 2003. Proteins of multiple classes may participate in nongenomic steroid actions. Exp Biol Med (Maywood) 228:1272-1281.

Welshons WV, Thayer KA, Judy BM, Taylor JA, Curran EM, Vom Saal FS. 2003. Large effects from small exposures. I. Mechanisms for endocrine-disrupting chemicals with estrogenic activity. Environ Health Perspect 111:994-1006.

Wozniak AL, Bulayeva NN, Watson CS. 2005. Xenoestrogens at picomolar to nanomolar concentrations trigger membrane estrogen receptor-α-mediated Ca2+ fluxes and prolactin release in GH3/B6 pituitary tumor cells. Environ Health Perspect 113:431-439.

Yunginger JW, Reed CE, O'Connell EJ, Melton LJ III, O'Fallon WM, Silverstein MD. 1992. A community-based study of the epidemiology of asthma. Incidence rates, 1964-1983. Am Rev Respir Dis 146:888-894.

Zaitsu M, Narita S, Lambert KC, Grady JJ, Estes DM, Curran EM, et al. 2006. Estradiol activates mast cells via a non-genomic estrogen receptor-α and calcium influx. Mol Immunol doi:10.1016/j.molimm.2006.09.030 [Online 3 November, 2006].

Maternal Bisphenol A Exposure Promotes the Development of Experimental Asthma in Mouse Pups

Terumi Midoro-Horiuti[1,2], Ruby Tiwari[1], Cheryl S. Watson[2], and Randall M. Goldblum[1,2]

[1]Department of Pediatrics, Child Health Research Center;

and [2]Department of Biochemistry and Molecular Biology, University of Texas Medical Branch, Galveston, TX, USA

Abstract

Background: We recently reported that various environmental estrogens induce mast cell degranulation and enhance IgE-mediated release of allergic mediators *in vitro*.

Objectives: We hypothesized that environmental estrogens would enhance allergic sensitization as well as bronchial inflammation and responsiveness. To test this hypothesis, we exposed fetal and neonatal mice to the common environmental estrogen bisphenol A (BPA) via maternal loading and assessed the pups' response to allergic sensitization and bronchial challenge. **Methods:** Female BALB/c mice received 10 μg/mL BPA in their drinking water from 1 week before impregnation to the end of the study. Neonatal mice were given a single 5 μg intraperitoneal dose of ovalbumin (OVA) with aluminum hydroxide on postnatal day 4 and 3% OVA by nebulization for 10 min on days 13, 14, and 15. Forty-eight hours after the last nebulization, we assessed serum IgE antibodies to OVA by enzyme-linked immunosorbent assay (ELISA) and airway inflammation and hyperresponsiveness by enumerating eosinophils in bronchoalveolar lavage fluid, whole-body barometric plethysmography, and a forced oscillation technique. **Results:** Neonates from BPA-exposed mothers responded to this "suboptimal" sensitization with higher serum IgE anti-OVA concentrations compared with those from unexposed mothers ($p < 0.05$), and eosinophilic inflammation in their airways was significantly greater. Airway responsiveness of the OVA-sensitized neonates from

BPA-treated mothers was enhanced compared with those from unexposed mothers ($p < 0.05$). **Conclusions:** Perinatal exposure to BPA enhances allergic sensitization and bronchial inflammation and responsiveness in a susceptible animal model of asthma.

Key words: airway hyperresponsiveness, asthma, bisphenol A, environmental estrogen, eosinophilia, experimental asthma, IgE, maternal exposure, perinatal sensitization.

Environ Health Perspect 118:273–277 (2010). doi:10.1289/ehp.0901259 available via *http://dx.doi.org/* [Online 5 October 2009]

References:

Adler A, Cieslewicz G, Irvin CG. 2004. Unrestrained plethysmography is an unreliable measure of airway responsiveness in BALB/c and C57BL/6 mice. J Appl Physiology 97:286-292.

Allam JP, Zivanovic O, Berg C, Gembruch U, Bieber T, Novak N. 2005. In search for predictive factors for atopy in human cord blood. Allergy 60:743-750.

Anderson SC, Poulsen KB. 2003. White blood cells. Anderson's Atlas of Hematology. Philadelphia: Lippincott Williams & Wilkins, 57-128.

Bulayeva NN, Watson CS. 2004. Xenoestrogen-induced ERK-1 and ERK-2 activation via multiple membrane-initiated signaling pathways. Environ Health Perspect 112:1481-1487.

Castro SM, Guerrero-Plata A, Suarez-Real G, Adegboyega PA,

Colasurdo GN, Khan AM, et al. 2006. Antioxidant treatment ameliorates respiratory syncytial virus-induced disease and lung inflammation. Am J Respir Crit Care Med 174:1361-1369.

Curran EM, Judy BM, Newton LG, Lubahn DB, Rottinghaus GE, MacDonald RS, et al. 2004. Dietary soy phytoestrogens and ERα signalling modulate interferon gamma production in response to bacterial infection. Clin Exp Immunol 135:219-225.

Dewailly É, Ayotte P, Bruneau S, Laliberte C, Muir DC, Norstrom RJ. 1993. Inuit exposure to organochlorines through the aquatic food chain in Arctic Quebec. Environ Health Perspect 101:618-620.

Dirtu AC, Roosens L, Geens T, Gheorghe A, Neels H, Covaci A. 2008. Simultaneous determination of bisphenol A, triclosan, and tetrabromobisphenol A in human serum using solid-phase extraction and gas chromatography-electron capture negative-ionization mass spectrometry. Anal Bioanal Chem 391:1175-1181.

Fedulov AV, Leme A, Yang Z, Dahl M, Lim R, Mariani TJ, et al. 2008. Pulmonary exposure to particles during pregnancy causes increased neonatal asthma susceptibility. Am J Respir Cell Mol Biol 38:57-67.

Fernandez MF, Arrebola JP, Taoufiki J, Navalon A, Ballesteros O, Pulgar R, et al. 2007. Bisphenol-A and chlorinated derivatives in adipose tissue of women. Reprod Toxicol 24:259-264.

Gern JE, Lemanske RF Jr, Busse WW. 1999. Early life origins of asthma. J Clin Invest 104:837-843.

Hamada K, Suzaki Y, Leme A, Ito T, Miyamoto K, Kobzik L, et al. 2007. Exposure of pregnant mice to an air pollutant aerosol increases asthma susceptibility in offspring. J Toxicol Environ Health A 70:688-695.

Holt PG, Jones CA. 2000. The development of the immune system during pregnancy and early life. Allergy 55:688-697.

Iwata M, Eshima Y, Kagechika H, Miyaura H. 2004. The endocrine disruptors nonylphenol and octylphenol exert direct effects on T cells to suppress Th1 development and enhance Th2 development. Immunol Lett 94:135-139.

Johnson CC, Ownby DR, Peterson EL. 1996. Parental history of atopic disease and concentration of cord blood IgE. Clin Exp Allergy 26:624-629.

Kabuto H, Amakawa M, Shishibori T. 2004. Exposure to bisphenol A during embryonic/fetal life and infancy increases oxidative injury and causes underdevelopment of the brain and testis in mice. Life Sci 74:2931-2940.

Kim YH, Kim CS, Park S, Han SY, Pyo MY, Yang M. 2003. Gender differences in the levels of bisphenol A metabolites in urine. Biochem Biophys Res Commun 312:441-448.

Kuroda N, Kinoshita Y, Sun Y, Wada M, Kishikawa N, Nakashima K, et al. 2003. Measurement of bisphenol A levels in human blood serum and ascitic fluid by HPLC using a fluorescent labeling reagent. J Pharm Biomed Anal 30:1743-1749.

Lambert KC, Curran EM, Judy BM, Milligan GN, Lubahn DB, Estes DM. 2005. Estrogen receptor α (ERα) deficiency in macrophages results in increased stimulation of CD4+ T cells while 17β-estradiol acts through ERα to increase IL-4 and GATA-3 expression in CD4+ T cells independent of antigen presentation. J Immunol 175:5716-5723.

Lee MH, Chung SW, Kang BY, Park J, Lee CH, Hwang SY, et al. 2003. Enhanced interleukin-4 production in CD4+ T cells and elevated immunoglobulin E levels in antigen-primed mice by bisphenol A and nonylphenol, endocrine disruptors: involvement of nuclear factor-AT and Ca2+. Immunology 109:76-86.

Leme AS, Hubeau C, Xiang Y, Goldman A, Hamada K, Suzaki Y, et al. 2006. Role of breast milk in a mouse model of maternal transmission of asthma susceptibility. J Immunol 176:762-769.

McCoy L, Redelings M, Sorvillo F, Simon P. 2005. A multiple cause-of-death analysis of asthma mortality in the United States, 1990-2001. J Asthma 42:757-763.

Nakano N, Nishiyama C, Yagita H, Koyanagi A, Akiba H, Chiba S, et al. 2009. Notch signaling confers antigen-presenting cell functions on mast cells. J Allergy Clin Immunol 123:74-81.

Narita S, Goldblum RM, Watson CS, Brooks EG, Estes DM, Curran EM, et al. 2007. Environmental estrogens induce mast cell degranulation and enhance IgE-mediated release of allergic mediators. Environ Health Perspect 115:48-52.

Ohshima Y, Yamada A, Tokuriki S, Yasutomi M, Omata N, Mayumi M. 2007. Transmaternal exposure to bisphenol A modulates the development of oral tolerance. Pediatr Res 62:60-64.

Padmanabhan V, Siefert K, Ransom S, Johnson T, Pinkerton J, Anderson L, et al. 2008. Maternal bisphenol-A levels at delivery: a looming problem? J Perinatol 28:258-263.

Prescott SL, Macaubas C, Holt BJ, Smallacombe TB, Loh R, Sly PD, et al. 1998. Transplacental priming of the human immune system to environmental allergens: universal skewing of initial T cell responses toward the Th2 cytokine profile. J Immunol 160:4730-4737.

Prescott SL, Macaubas C, Smallacombe T, Holt BJ, Sly PD, Holt PG. 1999. Development of allergen-specific T-cell memory in atopic and normal children. Lancet 353:196-200.

Sayed BA, Brown MA. 2007. Mast cells as modulators of T-cell responses. Immunol Rev 217:53-64.

Schonfelder G, Wittfoht W, Hopp H, Talsness CE, Paul M, Chahoud I. 2002. Parent bisphenol A accumulation in the human maternal-fetal-placental unit. Environ Health Perspect 110:A703-A707.

Shore SA, Rivera-Sanchez YM, Schwartzman IN, Johnston RA. 2003. Responses to ozone are increased in obese mice. J Appl Physiology 95:938-945.

Siegrist CA. 2001. Neonatal and early life vaccinology. Vaccine 19:3331-3346.

Solomon GM, Weiss PM. 2002. Chemical contaminants in breast milk: time trends and regional variability. Environ Health Perspect 110:A339-A347.

Sudowe S, Rademaekers A, Kolsch E. 1997. Antigen dose-dependent predominance of either direct or sequential switch in IgE antibody responses. Immunology 91:464-472.

Sun Y, Irie M, Kishikawa N, Wada M, Kuroda N, Nakashima K. 2004. Determination of bisphenol A in human breast milk by HPLC with column-switching and fluorescence detection. Biomed Chromatogr 18:501-507.

Tsukioka T, Brock J, Graiser S, Nguyen J, Nakazawa H, Makino T. 2003. Determination of trace amounts of bisphenol A in urine by negative-ion chemical-ionization-gas chromatography/mass spectrometry. Anal Sci 19:151-153.

Volkel W, Bittner N, Dekant W. 2005. Quantitation of bisphenol A and bisphenol A glucuronide in biological samples by high performance liquid chromatography-tandem mass spectrometry. Drug Metab Dispos 33:1748-1757.

Vollmer WM, Osborne ML, Buist AS. 1998. Twenty-year trends in the prevalence of asthma and chronic airflow obstruction in an HMO. Am J Respir Crit Care Med 157:1079-1084.

Wang SL, Lin CY, Guo YL, Lin LY, Chou WL, Chang LW. 2004. Infant exposure to polychlorinated dibenzo-*p*-dioxins, dibenzofurans and biphenyls (PCDD/Fs, PCBs)—correlation between prenatal and postnatal exposure. Chemosphere 54:1459-1473.

Watson CS, Gametchu B. 2001. Membrane estrogen and glucocorticoid receptors—implications for hormonal control of immune function and autoimmunity. Int Immunopharmacol 1:1049-1063.

Yang L, Hu Y, Hou Y. 2006. Effects of 17β-estradiol on the maturation, nuclear factor kappa B p65 and functions of murine spleen CD11c-positive dendritic cells. Mol Immunol 43:357-366.

Ye X, Kuklenyik Z, Needham LL, Calafat AM. 2005. Quantification of urinary conjugates of bisphenol A, 2,5-dichlorophenol, and 2-hydroxy-4-methoxybenzophenone in humans by online solid phase extraction-high performance liquid chromatography-tandem mass spectrometry. Anal Bioanal Chem 383:638-644.

Zaitsu M, Narita S, Lambert KC, Grady JJ, Estes DM, Curran EM, et al. 2007. Estradiol activates mast cells via a non-genomic estrogen receptor-α and calcium influx. Mol Immunol 44:1987-1995.

Gender-medicine aspects in allergology

E. Jensen-Jarolim, E. Untersmayr

Department of Pathophysiology, Center of Physiology, Pathophysiology and Immunology,

Medical University Vienna, Vienna, Austria

Abstract:

Despite the identical immunological mechanisms activating the release of mediators and consecutive symptoms in immediate-type allergy, there is still a clear clinical difference between female and male allergic patients. Even though the risk of being allergic is greater for boys in childhood, almost from adolescence onwards it seems to be a clear disadvantage to be a woman as far as atopic disorders are concerned. Asthma, food allergies and anaphylaxis are more frequently diagnosed in females. In turn, asthma and hay fever are associated with irregular menstruation. Pointing towards a role of sex hormones, an association of asthma and intake of contraceptives, and a risk for asthma exacerbations during pregnancy have been observed. Moreover, peri- and postmenopausal women were reported to increasingly suffer from asthma, wheeze and hay fever, being even enhanced by hormone replacement therapy. This may be on account of the recently identified oestradiol-receptor-dependent mast-cell activation. As a paradox of nature, women may even become hypersensitive against their own sex hormones, resulting in positive reactivity upon intradermal injection of oestrogen or progesterone. More importantly, this specific hypersensitivity is associated with recurrent miscarriages. Even though there is a striking gender specific bias in IgE-mediated allergic diseases, public awareness of this fact still remains minimal today.

References:

Almqvist C, Worm M, Leynaert B. Impact of gender on asthma in childhood and adolescence: a GA(2)LEN review. Allergy 2008; 63:47-57.

Association of asthma and hay fever with irregular menstruation. Thorax 2005; 60:445-450.

Balzano G, Fuschillo S, Melillo G, Bonini S. Asthma and sex hormones. Allergy 2001; 56:13-20.

Becklake MR, Kauffmann F. Gender differences in airway behaviour over the human life span. Thorax 1999; 54:1119-

1138.

Bender AE, Matthews DR. Adverse reactions to foods. Br J Nutr 1981; 46:403-407.

Benyamini Y, Leventhal EA, Leventhal H. Gender differences in processing information for making self-assessments of health. Psychosom Med 2000; 62:354-364.

Binkley KE, Davis AE III. Estrogendependent inherited angio-edema. Transfus Apher Sci 2003; 29:215-219.

Birrell SN, Butler LM, Harris JM, Buchanan G, Tilley WD. Disruption of androgen receptor signaling by synthetic progestins may increase risk of developing breast cancer. FASEB J 2007; 21:2285-2293.

Burr ML, Merrett TG. Food intolerance: a community survey. Br J Nutr 1983; 49:217-219.

Carroll KN, Gebretsadik T, Griffin MR, Dupont WD, Mitchel EF, Wu P, et al. Maternal asthma and maternal smoking are associated with increased risk of bronchiolitis during infancy. Pediatrics 2007; 119:1104-1112.

Chalubinski M, Kowalski ML. Endocrine disrupters—potential modulators of the immune system and allergic response. Allergy 2006; 61:1326-1335.

Chhabra SK. Premenstrual asthma. Indian J Chest Dis Allied Sci 2005; 47:109-116.

Ciray M, Mollard H, Duret M. Asthma and menstruation. Presse

Med 1938; 38:755-759.

Cocchiara R, Albeggiani G, Di Trapani G, Azzolina A, Lampiasi N, Rizzo F, et al. Oestradiol enhances in vitro the histamine release induced by embryonic histamine releasing factor (EHRF) from uterine mast cells. Hum Reprod 1992; 7:1036-1041.

Cocchiara R, Albeggiani G, Di Trapani G, Azzolina A, Lampiasi N, Rizzo F, et al. Modulation of rat peritoneal mast cell and human basophil histamine release by estrogens. Int Arch Allergy Appl Immunol 1990; 93:192-197.

Coogan PF, Palmer JR, et al. 2009. Body mass index and asthma incidence in the Black Women's Health Study. J Allergy Clin Immunol 123(1): 89-95.

Cutolo M, Capellino S, Sulli A, Serioli B, Secchi ME, Villaggio B, et al. Estrogens and autoimmune diseases. Ann N Y Acad Sci 2006; 1089:538-547.

Da Silva JA. Sex hormones and glucocorticoids: interactions with the immune system. Ann N Y Acad Sci 1999; 876:102-117.

Daeron M. Fc receptor biology. Annu Rev Immunol 1997; 15:203-234.

Dean NL. Perimenstrual asthma exacerbations and positioning of leukotriene-modifying agents in asthma management guidelines. Chest 2001; 120:2116-2117.

Dewyea VA, Nelson MR, Martin BL. Asthma in pregnancy. Allergy Asthma Proc 2005; 26:323-325.

Dijkstra A, Howard TD, Vonk JM, Ampleford EJ, Lange LA, Bleecker ER, et al. Estrogen receptor 1 polymorphisms are associated with airway hyperresponsiveness and lung function decline, particularly in female subjects with asthma. J Allergy Clin Immunol 2006; 117:604-611.

Dunn Galvin A, Hourihane JO, Frewer L, Knibb RC, Oude Elberink JN, Klinge I. Incorporating a gender dimension in food allergy research: a review. Allergy 2006; 61:1336-1343.

Eisenberg SW, Cacciatore G, Klarenbeek S, Bergwerff AA, Koets AP. Influence of 17beta-oestradiol, nortestosterone and dexamethasone on the adaptive immune response in veal calves. Res Vet Sci 2008; 84: 199-205.

Ford ES, Mannino DM, Homa DM, Gwynn C, Redd SC, Moriarty DG, et al. Self-reported asthma and health-related quality of life: findings from the behavioral risk factor surveillance system. Chest 2003; 123:119-127.

Furuichi K, Rivera J, Isersky C. The receptor for immunoglobulin E on rat basophilic leukemia cells: effect of ligand binding on receptor expression. Proc Natl Acad Sci USA 1985; 82:1522-1525.

Geiger E, Magerstaedt R, Wessendorf JH, Kraft S, Hanau D, Bieber T. IL-4 induces the intracellular expression of the alpha chain of the high-affinity receptor for IgE in in vitro-generated dendritic cells. J Allergy Clin Immunol 2000; 105:150-156.

Gluck JC. The change of asthma course during pregnancy. Clin Rev Allergy Immunol 2004; 26:171-180.

Gomez Real F, Svanes C, Bjornsson EH, Franklin KA, Gislason D, Gislason T, et al. Hormone replacement therapy, body mass index and asthma in perimenopausal women: a cross sectional survey. Thorax 2006; 61:34-40.

Grimaldi CM. Sex and systemic lupus erythematosus: the role of the sex hormones estrogen and prolactin on the regulation of autoreactive B cells. Curr Opin Rheumatol 2006; 18:456-461.

Gruijthuijsen YK, Grieshuber I, Stocklinger A, Tischler U, Fehrenbach T, Weller MG, et al. Nitration enhances the allergenic potential of proteins. Int Arch Allergy Immunol 2006; 141:265-275.

Haggerty CL, Ness RB, Kelsey S, Waterer GW. The impact of estrogen and progesterone on asthma. Ann Allergy Asthma Immunol 2003; 90:284-291; quiz 291-283, 347.

Hanania NA, Belfort MA. Acute asthma in pregnancy. Crit Care Med 2005; 33:S319-S324.

Hantusch B, Schöll I, Harwanegg C, Krieger S, Becker WM, Spitzauer S, et al. Affinity determinations of purified IgE and IgG antibodies against the major pollen allergens Phl p 5a and Betv 1a: discrepancy between IgE and IgG binding strength. Immunol Lett 2005; 97:81-89.

Harnish DC, Albert LM, Leathurby Y, Eckert AM, Ciarletta A, Kasaian M, et al. Beneficial effects of estrogen treatment in the HLA-B27 transgenic rat model of inflammatory bowel disease. Am J Physiol Gastrointest Liver Physiol 2004; 286:G118-G125.

Hendler I, Schatz M, Momirova V, Wise R, Landon M, Mabie W, et al. Association of obesity with pulmonary and nonpulmonary complications of pregnancy in asthmatic women. Obstet Gynecol 2006; 108:77-82.

Itsekson AM, Seidman DS, Zolti M, Lazarov A, Carp HJ. Recurrent pregnancy loss and inappropriate local immune response to sex hormones. Am J Reprod Immunol 2007; 57:160-165.

Jaakkola JJ, Ahmed P, Ieromnimon A, Goepfert P, Laiou E, Quansah R, et al. Preterm delivery and asthma: a systematic review and meta-analysis. J Allergy Clin Immunol 2006; 118:823-830.

Jakobsen CG, Bodtger U, Poulsen LK, Roggen EL. Vaccination for birch pollen allergy: comparison of the affinities of specific immunoglobulins E, G1 and G4 measured by surface plasmon resonance. Clin Exp Allergy 2005; 35:193-198.

Jansen JJ, Kardinaal AF, Huijbers G, Vlieg-Boerstra BJ, Martens BP, Ockhuizen T. Prevalence of food allergy and intolerance in the adult Dutch population. J Allergy Clin Immunol 1994; 93:446-456.

Jiang YA, Zhang YY, Luo HS, Xing SF. Mast cell density and the context of clinicopathological parameters and expression of p185, estrogen receptor, and proliferating cell nuclear antigen in gastric carcinoma. World J Gastroenterology 002; 8:1005-1008.

Kinet JP. The high-affinity IgE receptor (Fc epsilon RI): from physiology to pathology. Annu Rev Immunol 1999; 17:931-972.

Kiriyama K, Sugiura H, Uehara M. Premenstrual deterioration of skin symptoms in female patients with atopic dermatitis. Dermatology 2003; 206:110-112.

Lang TJ. Estrogen as an immunomodulator. Clin Immunol 2004; 113:224-230.

Lenoir RJ. Severe acute asthma and the menstrual cycle. Anaesthesia 1987; 42:1287-1290.

Lovik M, Namork E, Faeste C, Egaas E. The Norwegian National Reporting System and Register of Severe Allergic Reactions to Food. Clinical Immunology and Allergy in Medicine. Marone G, editor. Napoli: JGC Publishers, 2003:461-466.

Ma LJ, Guzman EA, DeGuzman A, Muller HK, Walker AM, Owen LB. Local cytokine levels associated with delayed-type hypersensitivity responses: modulation by gender, ovariectomy, and estrogen replacement. J Endocrinol 2007; 193:291-297.

Maleki SJ, Chung SY, Champagne ET, Raufman JP. The effects of roasting on the allergenic properties of peanut proteins. J Allergy Clin Immunol 2000; 106:763-768.

Maleki SJ, Kopper RA, Shin DS, Park CW, Compadre CM, Sampson H, et al. Structure of the major peanut allergen Ara h 1 may protect IgE-binding epitopes from degradation. J Immunol 2000; 164:5844-5849.

Maranghi F, Rescia M, Macri C, Di Consiglio E, De Angelis G, Testai E, et al. Lindane may modulate the female reproductive development through the interaction with ER-beta: an in vivo-in vitro approach. Chem Biol Interact 2007; 169:1-14.

Martinez-Moragon E, Plaza V, Serrano J, Picado C, Galdiz JB, Lopez-Vina A, et al. Near-fatal asthma related to menstruation. J Allergy Clin Immunol 2004; 113:242-244.

Masuch GI, Franz JT, Schoene K, Musken H, Bergmann KC. Ozone increases group 5 allergen content of Lolium perenne. Allergy 1997; 52: 874-875.

Metcalfe D. Food allergy in adults. Chapter 10 from Food Allergy: Adverse Reactions to Foods and Food Additives, 3rd ed. USA: Blackwell Sciences, 2003:36-143.

Metzger H. The receptor with high affinity for IgE. Immunol Rev 1992; 125:37-48.

Mitchell VL, Gershwin LJ. Progesterone and environmental tobacco smoke act synergistically to exacerbate the development of allergic asthma in a mouse model. Clin Exp Allergy 2007; 37:276-286.

Möhrenschlager M, Schäfer T, Huss-Marp J, Eberlein-König B, Weidinger S, Ring J, et al. The course of eczema in children aged 5-7 years and its relation to atopy: differences between boys and girls. Br J Dermatology 2006; 154:505-513.

Moneret-Vautrin DA, Morisset M. Adult food allergy. Curr Allergy Asthma Rep 2005; 5:80-85.

Narita S, Goldblum RM, Watson CS, Brooks EG, Estes DM, Curran EM, et al. Environmental estrogens induce mast cell degranulation and enhance IgE-mediated release of allergic mediators. Environ Health Perspect 2007; 115:48-52.

Nicovani S, Rudolph MI. Estrogen receptors in mast cells from arterial walls. Biocell 2002; 26:15-24.

Novak N, Tepel C, Koch S, Brix K, Bieber T, Kraft S. Evidence for a differential expression of the FcepsilonRIgamma chain in dendritic cells of atopic and nonatopic donors. J Clin Invest 2003; 111:1047-1056.

Quarto R, Kinet JP, Metzger H. Coordinate synthesis and degradation of the alpha-, beta- and gamma-subunits of the receptor for immunoglobulin E. Mol Immunol 1985; 22:1045-1051.

Rahimi R, Nikfar S, Abdollahi M. Meta-analysis finds use of inhaled corticosteroids during pregnancy safe: a systematic meta-analysis review. Hum Exp Toxicol 2006; 25:447-452

Regal JF, Fraser DG, Weeks CE, Greenberg NA. Dietary phytoestrogens have anti-inflammatory activity in a guinea pig model of asthma. Proc Soc Exp Biol Med 2000; 223:372-378.

Riffo-Vasquez Y, Ligeiro de Oliveira AP, Page CP, Spina D, Tavares-de-Lima W. Role of sex hormones in allergic inflammation in mice. Clin Exp Allergy 2007; 37:459-470.

Roby RR, Richardson RH, Vojdani A. Hormone allergy. Am J Reprod Immunol 2006; 55:307-313.

Salam MT, Wenten M, Gilliland FD. Endogenous and exogenous sex steroid hormones and asthma and wheeze in young women. J Allergy Clin Immunol 2006; 117:1001-1007.

Schäfer T, Bohler E, Ruhdorfer S, Weigl L, Wessner D, Heinrich J, et al. Epidemiology of food allergy/food intolerance in adults: associations with other manifestations of atopy. Allergy 2001; 56:1172-1179.

Schöll I, Kalkura N, Shedziankova Y, Bergmann A, Verdino P, Knittelfelder R, et al. Dimerization of the major birch pollen allergen Bet v 1 is important for its in vivo IgE-crosslinking potential in mice. J Immunol 2005; 175:6645-6650.

Searing DA, Zhang Y, et al. 2010. Decreased serum vitamin D levels in children with asthma are associated with increased corticosteroid use. J Allergy Clin Immunol 125(5): 995-1000.

Siroux V, Curt F, Oryszczyn MP, Maccario J, Kauffmann F. Role of gender and hormone-related events on IgE, atopy, and eosinophils in the Epidemiological Study on the Genetics and Environment of Asthma, bronchial hyperresponsiveness and atopy. J Allergy Clin Immunol 2004; 114:491-498.

Skobeloff EM, Spivey WH, Silverman R, Eskin BA, Harchelroad F, Alessi TV. The effect of the menstrual cycle on asthma presentations in the emergency department. Arch Intern Med 1996; 156:1837-1840.

Spanos C, el-Mansoury M, Letourneau R, Minogiannis P, Greenwood J, Siri P, et al. Carbachol-induced bladder mast cell activation: augmentation by estradiol and implications for interstitial cystitis. Urology 1996; 48:809-816.

Sterk AR, Ishizaka T. Binding properties of IgE receptors on normal mouse mast cells. J Immunol 1982; 128:838-843.

Stygar D, Masironi B, Eriksson H, Sahlin L. Studies on estrogen receptor (ER) alpha and beta responses on gene regulation in peripheral blood leukocytes in vivo using selective ER agonists. J Endocrinol 2007; 194:101-119.

Suzuki K, Hasegawa T, Sakagami T, Koya T, Toyabe S, Akazawa K, et al. Analysis of perimenstrual asthma based on question-naire surveys in Japan. Allergol Int 2007; 56:249-255.

Svanes C, Real FG, Gislason T, Jansson C, Jogi R, Norrman E, et al. Association of asthma and hay fever with irregular menstruation. Thorax 2005; 60:445-450.

Tata LJ, Lewis SA, McKeever TM, Smith CJ, Doyle P, Smeeth L, et al. A comprehensive analysis of adverse obstetric and pediatric complications in women with asthma. Am J Respir Crit Care Med 2007; 175:991-997.

Temprano J and Mannino DM. 2009. The effect of sex on asthma control from the National Asthma Survey. J Allergy Clin Immunol 123(4): 854-860.

The British Dietetic Association. Paediatric group position statement on the use of soya protein for infants. J Fam Health Care 2003; 13:93.

The pill, breast cancer risk and your age. Mayo Clin Health Lett 2007; 25:4.

Thomas K, Herouet-Guicheney C, Ladics G, Bannon G, Cockburn A, Crevel R, et al. Evaluating the effect of food processing on the potential human allergenicity of novel proteins: international workshop report. Food Chem Toxicol 2007; 45:1116-1122.

Vasiadi M, Kempuraj D, Boucher W, Kalogeromitros D, Theoharides TC. Progesterone inhibits mast cell secretion. Int J Immunopathol Pharmacol 2006; 19:787-794.

Vliagoftis H, Dimitriadou V, Boucher W, Rozniecki JJ, Correia I, Raam S, et al. Estradiol augments while tamoxifen inhibits rat mast cell secretion. Int Arch Allergy Immunol 1992; 98:398-409.

Vrieze A, Postma DS, Kerstjens HA. Perimenstrual asthma: a syndrome without known cause or cure. J Allergy Clin Immunol 2003; 112:271-282.

Watson HG. Sex hormones and thrombosis. Semin Hematol 2007; 44:98-105.

Webb LM, Lieberman P. Anaphylaxis: a review of 601 cases. Ann Allergy Asthma Immunol 2006; 97:39-43.

Wizeman TM, Pardue ML. Exploring the biological contributions to human health: does sex matter? Institute of Medicine (IOM). Washington, D.C.: National Academic Press, 2003.

Young E, Stoneham MD, Petruckevitch A, Barton J, Rona R. A population study of food intolerance. Lancet 1994; 343:1127-1130.

Zaitsu M, Narita S, Lambert KC, Grady JJ, Estes DM, Curran EM, et al. Estradiol activates mast cells via a non-genomic estrogen receptor-alpha and calcium influx. Mol Immunol 2007; 44:1977-1985.

Zhang, Z, Lai HJ, et al. 2010. Early childhood weight status in relation to asthma development in high-risk children. J Allergy Clin Immunol 126(6): 1157-1162.

Zhao XJ, McKerr G, Dong Z, Higgins CA, Carson J, Yang ZQ, et al. Expression of oestrogen and progesterone receptors by mast cells alone, but not lymphocytes, macrophages or other immune cells in human upper airways. Thorax 2001; 56:205-211.

Chapter 4: SKIN TESTING AND ALLERGY VACCINE
References:

American Lung Association. Epidemiology and Statistics Unit, Best Practices And Program Services. Trends in Asthma Morbidity and Mortality, February 2002.

American Lung Association. Trends in Morbidity and Mortality. January 2001.

Asthma Prevalence, Health Care Use, and Mortality, 2000-2001, National Center for Health Statistics, Centers for Disease Control and Prevention.

CDC. Surveillance for Asthma – United States, 1980-1990. Morbidity and Mortality Weekly Report. 2002; 51(SS01): 1-13.

CDC. Surveillance for Asthma – United States, 1980-1990. Morbidity and Mortality Weekly Report. Surveillance Summaries, March 29, 2002.

CDC. Surveillance for asthma: United States, 1960-1995.

Morbidity and Mortality Weekly Report. 1998; 47(55-1): 1-28.

Des Roches A, Paradis L, Menardo IL, Bouges S, Daures J-P, Bousquet J. Immunotherapy with a standardized Dermato-phygoides pteronyssinus extract, VI: specific immunotherapy prevents the onset of new sensitization in children. J Allergy Clin Immunol. 1997; 99:450-453.

Di Rienzo V, et al. Post-marketing survey on the safety of sublingual immunotherapy in children below the age of 5 years. Clin Exp Allergy 2005; 35:560-564.

Evans, R. Asthma among Minority Children: A Growing Problem. Chest (1192) 101(6): 368S-71.

Fiocchi A, Pajno G, La Grutta S, Pezzuto F, Incorvaia C, Sensi L, Marcucci F, Frati F. Safety of sublingual-swallow immuno-therapy in children aged 3 to 7 years. Ann Allergy Asthma Immunol. 2005 Sep; 95(3):254-8.

Harold Nelson. Efficacy and safety of allergen immunotherapy in children, Ann Allergy Asthma Immunol. 2006; 96(Supply 1): S2-S5.

Martinez FD, Wright AL, Taussig LM, et al.: Asthma and wheezing in the first six years of life, New England Journal of Medicine. 332:133-138, 1995.

Möller C, Dreborg S, Ferdousi HA, et al. Pollen immunotherapy reduces the development of asthma in children with seasonal rhinoconjunctivitis (the PAT-Study). J Allergy Clin Immunol. 2002; 109:251-256.

National Center for Health Statistics. Raw Data from the National Health Interview Survey, U.S., 1997-1999. Analysis by the American Lung Association Best Practices Division, using SPSS and SUDAAN software.

National Heart, Lung, and Blood Institute. "Morbidity & Mortality: 2002 Chart Book on Cardiovascular, Lung, and Blood Diseases," National Institutes of Health, May 2002.

Pajno GB, Barberio G, De Luca FR, Morabito LO, Parmiani S. Prevention of new sensitizations in asthmatic children monosensitized to house dust mite by specific immunotherapy: a six-year follow-up study. Clin Exp Allergy. 2001; 31:1392-1397.

Purello-D'Ambrosio F, Gangemi S, Merendino RA, et al. Prevention of new sensitizations in monosensitized subjects submitted to specific immunotherapy or not: a retrospective study. Clin Exp Allergy. 2001; 31:1295-1302.

Roberts G, et al. Grass pollen immunotherapy as an effective therapy of childhood seasonal allergic asthma, J Allergy Clin Immunol. 2006; 117:26-8.

United States. Centers for Disease Control. Forecasted State – Specific Estimates of Self-Reported Asthma Prevalence – 1998. Morbidity and Mortality. (Dec. 4, 1998) 47:1022-1025.

Sensitization and immune cells response to allergen immunotherapy

Norman PS. 2004. Immunotherapy: 1999-2004. J Allergy Clin Immunol 113(6): 1013-1023.

Mast cell and basophil degranulation products

Simons FER, Frew AJ, et al. 2007. Risk assessment in anaphy-laxis: Current and future approaches. J Allergy Clin Immunol 120(1): S2-S24.

Chapter 5: MEDICATION THERAPY AND TREATMENT TECHNIQUES

www.orthomed.org

INDEX

A

AAAAI. *See* American Academy
    of Allergy, Asthma and
    Immunology
Acute conjunctivitis Nos, 93*t*
Acute ethmoidal sinusitis, 85*t*
Acute frontal sinusitis, 83*t*
Acute maxillary sinusitis, 81*t*
Acute sinusitis, other, 89*t*
Acute sphenoidal sinusitis, 87*t*
Adjuvant immunotherapy, 50–51
Adult-onset allergies
    estrogen dominance and,
        42, 74
    skin testing and, 42
    in women, 47–48
Adult-onset nasal symptoms, 2–3
Adult-onset rhinitis
    estrogen dominance and, 74
    perennial non-allergic
        rhinitis (PNAR) and, 74
Allergen immunotherapy (AIT)
    anaphylactic reaction, 44–
        46, 57, 61
    low-dose therapy, 57
    menstrual cycle and, 45–46
    patient testing, 57
    peripheral T cell tolerance,
        60
    sensitization, immune cells
        response, 136
    skin test reactivity and, 46,
        56–57

    summary of effects, 60
Allergen sensitization, reaction
    cascade, 55–56, 55*d*
Allergic conjunctivitis
    defined, 1
    treatment, 69
Allergic rhinitis, 32
    defined, 1
    due to pollen, 77*t*
    orthomolecular approach,
        71–72
    prevalence, 50
    seasonal *vs.* chronic, 50
Allergic rhinitis impact on asthma
    (ARIA), 32
Allergic rhinitis Nec, 78*t*
Allergic rhinitis Nos, 79*t*
Allergy categories, 1
Allergy theory, 37
Allergy vaccine, 49–50, 134–136
American Academy of Allergy,
    Asthma and Immunology
    (AAAAI), 29
Antigen-presenting cell (APC), 33
Antihistamines, 34–36
Antioxidants, 71–72
APC. *See* Antigen-presenting cell
ARIA. *See* Allergic rhinitis impact
    on asthma
Asthma, 32
    menstrual cycle and, 100–
        101
    premenstrual exacerbation

(PMA) of, 98–99
Atopic dermatitis (eczema), 32
Atopic diseases
    CDC reports, 39
    estrogen epidemic and, 40
    pathophysiology, 29d, 32,
        55–56, 55d, 62d, 73
Atopic march, 32

B

Basophil, activation products, 59t,
    137
Beclomethasone, 53
Benign prostatic hypertrophy
    (BPH), 9, 19
Benign tumors, 9, 19–20
Birth control pills, 15
BPH. See Benign prostatic
    hypertrophy
Breast cancer, estrogen,
    progesterone receptors,
    20–21
Budesonide, 26

C

Cancer, estrogens, 20
CD4+ T-cell, CD8+ T-cell, 60
Childhood allergies
    acute sinusitis, 32–33
    allergy theory, 37
    beclomethasone for, 53
    chronic sinusitis, 32
    food allergies, 32
    genetics and, 31
    high-dose sublingual
        immunotherapy (SLIT),
        52–53

specific immunotherapy
    (SIT), 53–54
sublingual immunotherapy
    (SLIT), 51–52
Chronic allergic conjunctivitis Nec,
    5–6, 95t
Chronic conjunctivitis Nos, 94t
Chronic ethmoidal sinusitis, 86t
Chronic frontal sinusitis, 84t
Chronic maxillary sinusitis, 82t
Chronic rhinitis, 80t
Chronic sinusitis Ned, 90t
Chronic sinusitis Nos, 92t
Chronic sphenoidal sinusitis, 88t
Ciclesonide, 36
Combination therapy, 36, 68–69,
    73
Copper
    estrogens and, 19
    thyroid function and, 19

E

Eczema. See Atopic dermatitis
Endocrine-disrupting chemicals
    (EDCs), 70–71
Endogenous estrogens, 6–7
Endogenous hormone production
    cascade, 8–10, 8d
Environmental Health
    Perspectives, 40
Eosinophil, 35, 56
Eosinophilic cationic protein (ECP),
    56
Estradiol, 40–41, 101–108
Estrogen receptor-alpha (ER-
    alpha), 40, 74
Estrogenic chemicals, allergic
    diseases, 21

Estrogen/progesterone imbalance, symptoms, 23–27

Estrogens
cancer and, 20
copper and, 19
endogenous, men, 6–7
environmental, 41–42
estrogen dominance, 7–13, 8d, 22, 43–44, 74
estrogen, progesterone cycle, 16d

F

FC epsilon receptor 1 (FC$_E$R1), 33–34
Fluticasone, 36
Food allergy, 32

G

Gender-medicine aspects, 121–134
Gene-environmental interactions, 31

H

Hay fever, 50
HCUP. *See* Healthcare Cost and Utilization Project
Health care providers, 1–2, 73
Healthcare Cost and Utilization Project (HCUP), 97
High-dose sublingual immunotherapy (SLIT), 52–53
Histamine, 34–35
Hormone imbalance

laboratory workup, 27
types, 27
Hormone Imbalance Syndrome: America's Silent Plague - Uncovering the Roots of the Obesity Epidemic and Common Diseases (Tano), 48, 74
Hygiene hypothesis, 31
Hypothyroidism, 18

I

IgM, IgE, 33–34
IgA, IgG4, 57
IL-4, IL-5, IL-13, 56
IL-10, 57
Interferon-γ, 60
Immunotherapy. *See* Allergen immunotherapy
Insulin resistance, 7–10, 8d

L

Laboratory workup, 27
Leptin resistance, 8d, 9
Leukotriene C4 (LTC4), 35, 40
Leukotriene receptor antagonist (LTRA), 35–36, 98–99
Levothyroxine, 18
LTC4. *See* Leukotriene C4
LTRA. *See* Leukotriene receptor antagonist

M

Macromedicine diagram, 8d
Major Basic Protein (MBP), 56
Mast cells, 137

activation products, 59*t*
degranulation causes, 41–
    42, 74
environmental estrogens
    and, 109–121
estradiol activation, 40–41,
    101–108
estrogens and, 40–48
Maternal bisphenol A (BPA)
    exposure, 113–115
Medication treatment, 49–51
    skin testing and, 56–57
Men, endogenous estrogens, 6–7
Menstrual cycle, allergen
    immunotherapy (AIT), 45–46
Montelukast, 35

N

Nasal corticosteroids (NCSs), 36
    effective techniques, 66–67
    sequence, optimal
        combination, 68–69
Nasal sprays, sequence, 68–69
NCS. *See* Nasal corticosteroids
Non-allergic rhinitis, defined, 1
Nutritional supplements, 43,
    71–72

O

Obesity, 6, 7–10, 8*d,* 39, 47–48, 74
Orthomolecular therapy, 70–72
Oxymetazoline, 1

P

Patient education, 73–74
Pauling, Linus, 70

Perennial non-allergic rhinitis
    (PNAR), 47, 63–64, 68–69
Phenylephrine, 2
Phytoestrogens, 22, 42–43
PMA. *See* Premenstrual
    exacerbations of asthma
PMDD. *See* Premenstrual
    dysphoric disorder
PMS. *See* Premenstrual syndrome
    (PMS)
PNAR. *See* Perennial non-allergic
    rhinitis
Postnasal drip, 2
Prednisone, 36
Pregnancy, progesterone
    deficiency, 14–15
Premenstrual dysphoric disorder
    (PMDD), 17
Premenstrual exacerbations of
    asthma (PMA), 98–99
Premenstrual syndrome (PMS), 17
Progesterone deficiency, 7–10, 8*d*
    adult onset, 15–18, 16*d*
    consequences, 14–15
    pregnancy and, 14–15
    thyroid function and, 18
    women, 15–18
Progesterone deficiency/estrogen
    dominance, 10–13
Progesterone, estrogen cycle, 16*d*
Progesterone/estrogen imbalance
    effects, women, 13–14
    symptoms, 23–27
Prostaglandins, 35–36

R

RBL-2H3, definition, 97–98
Reactive airway disease, 32

Rebound nasal congestion, 1
Respiratory syncytial virus (RSV) infection, 32
Rhinitis medicamentosa, 1
RSV. *See* Respiratory syncytial virus infection

S

Saline nasal sprays, 64–65. *See also* Nasal corticosteroids
Science, 70
Self-medication, 1, 35–36
Serotonin, 9
Sinusitis, defined, 1
Skin testing
    adult-onset allergies and, 42
    allergen immunotherapy (AIT) and, 46, 56–57
    allergy vaccine and, 134–136
    medication treatment, 56–57
    variables, 99–100
SLIT. *See* Sublingual immunotherapy
Specific immunotherapy (SIT), 53–54
Steroids, 35
Sublingual immunotherapy (SLIT), 51–52

T

T3, T4 thyroid hormone, 10, 18
Tano, Benoit, 48, 74
TGF-β, TGF-Beta, 57
Th0, Th1, Th2 cells, 33
Thyroid function, 18–19
TNF-α

T-regulatory cell cytokines, 61
Triamcinolone, 36
TSH, 18

U

University of Texas Medical Branch (UTMB), 40–42

W

Women
    atopic disease prevalence and, 74
    endogenous estrogens and, 6–7
    estrogens, benign tumors, 19–20
    obesity, comorbidities, 74
    progesterone deficiency, 15–18, 16*d*
    progesterone/estrogen imbalance effects, 13–14
    xenoestrogens and, 6

X

Xenoestrogens, 6, 22, 42–43

ABOUT THE AUTHOR

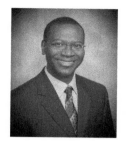

Benoît Tano, M.D., Ph.D.

Dr. Tano is currently a clinical associate professor of medicine with specialization in allergy and clinical immunology at the University of North Dakota School of Medicine and Health Sciences and is employed full-time as an allergist with the Altru Health System in Grand Forks, North Dakota.

Prior to joining Altru and UND, Dr. Tano completed a Ph.D. degree in economics at the State University of New York at Albany, with specialization in econometrics and labor economics (1988), and taught economics at the University of Toledo in Ohio (1988-1995). He then entered medical school and completed his M.D. degree at the Medical College of Ohio in 1999, followed by a three-year residency training in internal medicine at the Ohio State University Medical Center (1999-2002). In 2002, he engaged in a two-year fellowship training program in pharmacoeconomics and outcomes research, sponsored by GlaxoSmithKline and Ohio State University Medical Center (2002-2004). The research fellowship was followed by a clinical fellowship in allergy and immunology at the Johns Hopkins Asthma and Allergy Center in Baltimore, Maryland (July 2004-June 2006).

Dr. Tano is certified by the American Board of Internal Medicine, 2002, and by the American Board of Allergy and Immunology, 2006. Dr. Tano is a member of the American

Academy of Allergy, Asthma & Immunology, and the Academy of Anti-Aging and Regenerative Medicine.

CPSIA information can be obtained
at www.ICGtesting.com
Printed in the USA
LVHW04s2355011018
592105LV00001B/237/P